Laughter and Tears

FROM THE DIARIES WRITTEN BY THEIR LOVING SPOUSES

[signature]

'25 yrs of Research'

Laughter and Tears

FROM THE DIARIES WRITTEN
BY THEIR LOVING SPOUSES

by

MATT ALLEN *and* SALLY SILER

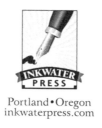

Portland•Oregon
inkwaterpress.com

Publisher: Inkwater Press | www.inkwaterpress.com

ISBN-13 978-1-62901-644-3 | ISBN-10 1-62901-644-6

1 3 5 7 9 10 8 6 4 2

Disclaimer

As the messenger (and author), I have compiled over two decades of health and medical data from medical doctors and scientists from around the globe. I pass this information along to readers. It is not intended as a diagnosis and/or a suggested treatment for a health condition. I mention supplements that I take as an example. They are effective with my body chemistry. Readers must consult their own health/medical professionals practicing in the area of their health conditions.

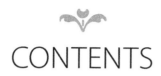

CONTENTS

INTRODUCTION

Alzheimer's disease (AD) is the most feared disease among adults polled in the United States—more than AIDS, cancer and heart disease. ("The Most Feared Terminal Disease," by Terry Lemerond, Nutrition and Alzheimer's, *Vitamin Retailer,* 2010.) The US has more than five million people with Alzheimer's at a cost of $209 billion per year. By 2050 the annual costs could soar to $1.1 trillion.

Currently, AD is the fifth leading cause of death in the US. The health of 35% of the caregivers of AD patients suffers, which compares to 19% among the caregivers of patients without dementia.

Since the year 2000, the death rate by heart disease has decreased by 14%. Meanwhile, the death rate by AD has increased by 89%. Of that number, 66% are women (World Health Organization statistics).

African Americans are twice as likely to become victims as white women. Hispanics are 1.5 times as likely to become victims as white women. These statistics were compiled by the Alzheimer's Association. The world death rates of AD per 100,000 population are as follows: Finland, 54; USA, 46; Canada, 36; Iceland, 34; Sweden, 32; Switzerland, 32; Norway, 30; Denmark, 30; the Netherlands, 29, and Belgium, 27. The lowest rates are in Africa, India, and South Asia. The Western diet increases the risk of AD. While world populations extend their life expectancy their death rates from AD increase. The average life expectancy in the nations with the highest death rates from AD is 82 years, whereas, the average life expectancy in the nations with the lowest death rates from AD is just over 67 years. The people of Africa, India, and South Asia do not live long enough to become victims of Alzheimer's disease!

As of January 2011, our nation finally placed research on Alzheimer's disease as a high priority—we were not the leader in the world. Research in AD has been a national priority in Australia, France, and the United Kingdom for years. Dementia costs the UK economy a billion pounds yearly, more than cancer and heart disease combined. Perhaps the unknown is what is most frightening to us human beings. Little is known, especially when you consider we've known about AD for over a hundred years.

ACKNOWLEDGMENTS

Ann Marie Paulsen, MD, was the answer to our prayers. She made sure I would survive. My family support kept me going ... daughters, sons-in-law, granddaughters, great-grandsons, and great-granddaughter. Persia Meyers, owner of the Ironwood Home, and her staff provided exceptional care for my wife. Hospice included harp music at the end. Pastor Paul Lyda, St. Matthew Lutheran Church, Beaverton, Oregon, was there for spiritual comfort.

–Matt Allen, author, messenger

Jesus was my rock, my guide through the journey. Greg and Bob, our sons, were there for me. Ellen Brandvoid, my sister, added support. Dave Woolery, caregiver at Dolphin Cove Care Home, cared for Fred when I could not.

–Sally Siler, co-author

Cover Photo: A scene of the surf at Westport, Washington. Compliments of professional photographer Ron Arel, of Westport.

DEDICATIONS—OUR SPOUSES

DEDICATED TO:
FREDERICK THAD SILER AKA "YOGI"
1936–2012 (76 YEARS OLD)

By Sally Siler

Fred was born in Cloudcroft, New Mexico. All that remains there now are giant mosquitoes. He was the youngest of five children and was taken care of by three doting older sisters and tolerated by one older brother. The whole family of six moved to Feather Falls, California, where they stayed in a two-bedroom house with dirt floors, an outhouse, and lots of laughter and great food. All the women were great cooks, really.

Fred's school years were spent in Oroville, California, with Dad working on the railroad and occasionally in the woods as a logger. In the summertime, Fred prowled the town with guys who became lifelong friends. They swam in Oroville Lake and did not don a pair of shoes or a shirt until September. School was not high on Fred's priority list. As a result, he had to repeat third grade. Fred's parents were refreshingly "old school" and did not question the opinion of his teacher.

High school was a time to shine, and shine he did. Fred took the Tigers to championships and charmed all the bobby-soxed girls that surrounded him. He definitely had "a way" that was like a magnet to all around him. The thing that made it so endearing was he did not realize it or exploit it. He graduated from sandlot ballgames into organized athletics and excelled. Now, Fred was catered to by more than just his sisters. As the quarterback and an indisputable leader of the team, he definitely received special treatment. During his junior year he would only eat hamburger patties and tomato soup for breakfast, lunch, and dinner. That is exactly what he was served by his mother and sisters at home and even by the caterers at the various sports banquets.

Although he lettered in football, baseball, and basketball, football rose to his favorite and so remained. He never lost a football game in high school. The winning streak continued in Yuba Junior College. Fred loved the game, and the game, in return, was good to him. If it had not been for football, his education would have ended at high school, if not in jail. He received a full scholarship from Yuba Junior College to the University of Oregon, thus forever to be known as a "Duck." The competition for positions became tougher. Oregon had the quarterback spot filled with a two-year varsity senior. Fred was red-shirted and moved to an end position. Always content in any situation, he made this change with his usual upbeat attitude. As a red-shirt he was on the 1958 Rose Bowl team, and he was so very proud of that. Those '58 players had such a tight comradeship with one another—their bond held for over three decades.

Len Casanova, the University of Oregon's coach, was a strong influence in Fred's life. His morals and values were not only preached, but lived. Oregon had gone to play Florida in that year, 1958. As the team entered a restaurant, the manager informed

Coach Casanova that the team was welcome, but the black player would have to eat in the kitchen. Coach Cas—aka the "Silver Fox"—took *all* his players and left. He was a real stand-up guy. During those Duck years Fred had a name change. Joe, a fellow player as well as a character like Fred, gave nicknames to some of the players. He dubbed Fred's roommate, John Wilcox, "Heckle" and Fred "Yogi." Joe had reasoned Yogi Berra was the ugliest man in baseball, thus Fred, the ugliest man in football, should have the same name. It was far from the truth, but the name stuck. Yogi was a character, a people magnet. The kind of guy everyone wanted to be around. Everyone wanted to sit at his table because they knew it would be the most fun.

I had transferred to the University of Oregon in my junior year. While I was sitting in the student union building at the beginning of the school year, I felt a tap on my shoulder. This adorable guy (Yogi) said, "Those are the eyes I'm going to marry." Unbeknownst to me at the time, he said similar lines to a lot of girls. But I was flattered and a little smitten.

"I'm sorry, Sally, it looks like your husband has Alzheimer's."

How can something so devastating have no shock value to me? My smart, witty, athletic husband with ... what? No connection. My rock would become a vegetable? It just did not seem possible that our memories of college, dates, births, trips, games, life would be ripped from him—from us—like pages from a book. Thus began my roller coaster ride from disbelief to despair.

When we met at college he was such a catch. Personality wrapped up inside an athletic body and social attitude ... one of "let's have fun." And fun we had ... from watching him on the football field to romantic moments by the river. Oh yeah, a few classes thrown in. That year of college was magical. We were together every moment possible. Because of dorm check—remember, this was 1959–60—I developed a plan to sneak out of the dorm undetected. And it worked. I took my roommate's feathered hat and positioned the feathers on the pillow to resemble my ponytail. Then out the window I went, crouching along the shrubs until I could dash across the street, catch a cab, and arrive at Yogi's.

The end of that year at the U of O found Yogi drafted into the Army and me pregnant. The Army sent Yogi to Germany for his duration to coach football for Special Services, which he did with the usual "Yogi gusto." Our baby was born in Bremerton, Washington, and did not meet his father until he was 18 months old. Every chance I got, I mentally played out the scenario of Yogi's return and loved every part of it.

We went from collegiate days to marriage, two kids, and a coaching career. Then those words:

"Sorry, Sally, it looks like your husband has Alzheimer's."

It was the year 2000. I took hold with the determination we would live through this together. Scared, but certain Yogi and I could do it. Not realizing "together" was gone forever, split right down the middle. Never having been around Alzheimer's, I could not accept the reality of life displayed by television and in nursing homes. My guy would not be anything like those images! They say that denial is a common reaction to devastating news. News like this not only brought out denial, but that denial stayed for the duration of the disease. I denied the onset of every new symptom. He looked so normal that I could not grasp he did not remember how to get to very familiar places. In my mind I felt sometimes it was "would not" rather than "could not." I found myself getting angry at him, but it was not him—it was Alzheimer's. But sadly, patience wears thin. Plus, I did not want him to not remember.

So, the first plan of attack was not to let him know. Suicide was a likely choice for him. He had said that many times. So we just kind of laughed at those "forgetful moments" that were coming closer and closer together. Ones like, "Where did I put my coffee? Did I already get the mail?" Those so-called "normal" moments most sixty-year-olds experience. We went on for a few months like this until it became visible enough to others for them to wonder and speculate. He was such a larger than life person in the small college town he taught and coached in. I just could not allow his legacy to be Alzheimer's.

As I watched the man I had always leaned on and followed grow more and more confused, I felt I had to protect his legacy and his dignity. He was known and loved by the whole area as a football coach, professor, friend, and a good time. The pictures I had seen on TV and books of Alzheimer patients seemed very remote to me ... what if it really did happen?

If you are reading this, please know there is no blueprint for caring for an Alzheimer's patient. There is absolutely no right or wrong way. Some methods and reactions work better than others. Redirecting Yogi's focus instead of just saying no worked well for me. If I said, "No, you can't go there to do that," he would just argue and fight (not physically). But if I said something like, "Okay, we'll go in just a minute. First, let's have a cup of coffee," he would forget all about it. Mistakes will be made, regrets will haunt you, but you're human and doing your best for the one you love.

My only sister lived in Tacoma, Washington, and had always wanted to live on the beach in the Grayland/Westport area. After talking with her and seeing the area and actually being quite numb at this point, I decided to be bold, take charge, and move. She decided the same. After all, we had started life together and would end life together. We would move far enough away to preserve Yogi's dignity in the minds and memories of those who once knew him. I put our home of 35 years up for sale. It sold within a week. Along with our border collie Zeke, Yogi and I headed north. We found and bought an ocean-front lot and started planning our new home. The move was necessary, I felt, to keep his dignity and memory intact; we could get through this thing with the ocean wind and waves as a background. I knew his friends and former players would find out sooner or later, but knowing with your head might be kinder than actually seeing it with your own eyes. By that time, Yogi was just relying on me and going along with the adventure I was telling him about. I, on the other hand, was relying heavily on prayer and direction from the Man above. He definitely supplied me with positive direction and assurance. The fact that the house sold so quickly and for more than the original asking price was like a flashing light pointing the way.

When we moved to Westport, Ellen—my only sister—also decided to move to the same small coastal community. So that would be an added blessing, one of support and family. Yogi and I stayed with them until we could find a rental to live in while our new home was being built. He enjoyed watching the contractor work. I can't honestly say the contractor enjoyed it, but he was so kind to Yogi that he would give him manual jobs to do, like cleaning up. Every time I watched him doing the sweeping it would tug at my heart. He used to do beautiful woodwork. He made Christmas presents. He made a bed out of pecan that is still gorgeous. He put in a wall of slanted pecan in the bedroom where the bed was placed. Now all he could do is pick up the nails. But he was happy to do it and I believe, or wanted to believe, he felt useful.

We made numerous trips to the big cities—Tacoma, Seattle, Olympia—to purchase house plans, permits, etc. This was all new to me, and unfortunately, it was to Yogi also. I am so grateful he wasn't aware of what used to be. There are two saving graces in this insidious disease: the patient does not know and is not in pain. While we were staying at Ellen's and finding a rental, Yogi had heard of the football program at Ocosta High School, part of a very small school district in Westport. He visited the facilities and was offered the job coaching there, which he took, naturally.

Looking for a rental went smoothly as I knew it was God's plan for us. I found a rental that I later dubbed our "surfer shack." It was cute, small, walking distance from the beach, and perfect for us at the time. Again, thank you, God. Yogi would go to practice and/or games while Zeke and I would go beach-combing. Kevin, the wrestling coach, became a friend to Yogi, as did everyone he met. As his mind slipped further and further, his football participation days came to an end. Kevin remained in contact and when the Oregon Ducks played the University of Washington Huskies in Seattle, he asked me if he could take "coach" up to the game. Seattle was about four hours away, so it would be a big excursion. I felt Yogi knew Kevin well enough and he loved his Ducks. Plus, Kevin would watch him carefully so he would not get lost. One worry was his "accidents." I told Kevin about the chances of Yogi wetting himself and said I would pack a couple of changes for him. Kevin said he was okay with that.

Hallucinations were very common during one of the phases. One afternoon he was looking out the front windows and became very agitated, saying Bobby, our youngest son, was out there and needed his help. Of course, Bobby was not there; he was deployed to Iraq. When I told him where Bobby was, he wanted to go there because Bobby "needed" him. Actually, that was probably close to being true. Later that day, I received an email from Bob and wanted to read it to Yogi. He was amazed Bobby was there, even though he did not really know where "there" was. It was a blessing for Yogi that he did not know of Bobby's three deployments. For me, it was very lonely not being able to share my worries, not having that shoulder to cry on, that rock to help hold me up.

So the day of the big rival game arrived. Yogi had quacked *a lot* about how the U of O was and always would be superior to the University of Washington, so they were all looking forward to it. I watched the game in my surfer shack. It was a barn-burner. Oregon won in the last few minutes and I knew Yogi was roaring and having a great ol' time. They came back late, but happy. When Kevin dropped off Yogi at our home, I asked Yogi how he enjoyed the game. He replied, "What game?" When people tell you to "live in the moment," I always remember that day and just exactly what it is to "live in the moment."

Our new ocean home was ready to occupy, two weeks short of one year. I called the moving van and arranged for all our things to be brought to the new location. Our possessions had been in storage for over a year. We placed all of the needed items in the house while Yogi watched or dusted. A zillion boxes were stored in the garage to be opened one by one. After all, we were both retired and could do it leisurely. Ha! Yogi would take a box into the house, unpack it, leave everything, empty box and all, right in the middle of the floor, then go get another box and do the same. So much for orderly arranging of household items. When I asked him to put the things away he did, bless his heart. (I can say that now, but to be perfectly honest I was not "blessing his heart" at all.) He would stash—and I do mean stash—them in the nearest empty cupboard. This meant towels would end up in the kitchen pan cupboard. I would spend the next few minutes diverting him to do something else and recruit my Ellen to assist me in "undo and redo."

When Ellen and I finally got to the new boxes in the garage we discovered some interesting items that had been packed away and stored for a year. I thought I had supervised all his packing, but I guess not. We opened one box and found one shoe, one very old, worn work shoe, with broken and cracked laces, dust, cobwebs, and a spider living in the toe. Only one person I know would deem that worthy of packing and preserving for a year.

The "two Davids" or "the twins" as Yogi would call them later, had always dreamed of opening a care home at the beach. They had vacationed here with Ellen and her husband, and both worked in Oregon as caregivers. They found a five-bedroom house they felt would be perfect. But they did not have sufficient funds to swing the deal. From the sale of our home in California, we had some extra cash in the bank. I offered to loan them the funds, interest free, with the stipulation there would be a room reserved for Yogi when it was time.

This phase in our life allowed me to work part time so I became a substitute teacher at the nearby elementary school. It was a welcome break for me even if it provided anxious moments when I returned not knowing what I would find. Luckily, nothing was at the dangerous point yet, and some events were rather comical. Laughter is such a relief. One day I came home after school and saw in my driveway and even spilling over to the neighbor's driveway, an assortment of emergency vehicles—a fire truck with firemen roaming about, an ambulance, and a fire chief's red car.

Needless to say my heart dropped until I saw *him*, my silly hubby, standing with a long blue raincoat on, an unlit cigar in his mouth, a rake in his hands, smiling goofily and waving at me. The first thing he said as I went to his side was, "I didn't do it … it was him!" He pointed to our neighbor, and he was correct. The neighbor had started burning some brush, and since we live right on the ocean, the wind caught it and started some of the dune grass smoldering. He was thoroughly enjoying all the commotion, just like a child would. His cigar smoking definitely didn't bring any danger, as he never could get it lit. If, by some chance, he managed to light it, his saliva would drown it out in no time. There he would be with his cigar, one at least five to six inches long, sticking out of his mouth with drool dripping off the end just puffing away. What a character.

There were things going on in our family Yogi was there for but not really comprehending. Our youngest son, Bob, was deployed to Iraq a couple of times. I silently watched all the news with worry, dread, and antidepressants. I felt as though Yogi thought it was a movie. Bob's camp was in Mosul when the mess hall got bombed. Yogi held me as I cried even though he did not know why. I wish now I had embraced the hug rather than resented the "all alone" feeling I had. I loved the hug, but it felt hollow, meaningless. During this stage (1 or 2 depending on which book you last consulted), I still had a small part of him. He was upright, confused, but still had control of his bodily functions. That was short-lived, however, and I did not appreciate what I had until it disintegrated. It started with "accidents." He would not be able to make it to the toilet in time and he had no control to hold it. There just wasn't enough time between "I have to go" and going. One nice afternoon, I took him down to the docks to have some coffee and watch a few crab boats come in. The gulls were eating the leftovers and the seals were playing in the water. I left him sitting on the bench while I went into one of the local gift shops with a large window so I could see him easily. I looked out and noticed him standing, looking very distressed. When I went out to him his pants were soaking wet. He said he was sorry he could not hold it. He was still able to realize embarrassment, which amazes me now as I did not realize he would not always register embarrassment. We went home and remedied the situation. There were some medications for this type of problem and the inevitable was delayed for a few months. But as I have come to realize, nothing solves the progression of Alzheimer's, it only postpones it. This gives you a few days, weeks, months of reprieve.

Here comes the first major problem. Actually, that's laughable—they're *all* large problems. Adult diapers, Depends, pads ... which one to choose and how to get them on? Yogi was still aware of dress and could easily find and choose his clothes and dress himself correctly. So introducing such a garment met with disgust, disdain, and refusal. After appealing to his... well, it's hard to say just *what* I appealed to, as common sense was all but gone, but I guess it was our relationship with each other because when I explained how much washing his "accidents" created, he consented to try the Depends. With that initial try, I removed all his boxer shorts and replaced them with Depends so when he got dressed that's all he could find. Presto!

Problem solved—at least *that* problem. When I had gone to the hospital supply store to buy Depends, I cried uncontrollably. I guess because I did not *know* that was a turning point for me, a sad facing of reality. The use of Depends had an effect on me also. I found any intimacy was very uncomfortable. It's very hard to get sexually close to one in diapers. As cruel as that sounds, it nevertheless is true.

The emergence of separate sleeping arrangements became a reality. I really believe it was harder on me than him. I sorely missed the closeness, and I still do. But there were some laughable moments too. One night the bells (I had them on every door) started to ring. It was the one on the front door. I jumped up to find him fully dressed, coat, hat, and all, on the front porch. When I inquired where he was going, he replied, "To the lodge for a cup of coffee." He said it so seriously and it was actually quite logical as we had vacationed many places that resembled this one and lodges were always an option. I had done my homework and read numerous books on the handling of AD decisions. Instead of saying "no" to him, I diverted his attention. "The lodge isn't open yet. See? It's all dark." Since it was around two in the morning, it *was* dark. "Let's go back in and I'll make you a cup and we can wait until it opens." When we got back in the house he took off his coat. I suggested we go to his room and rest while the coffee brewed. After taking off his shoes, we padded down the hallway to his room. There, I found his bed completely stripped, all sheets and blankets neatly folded and laying on the bed (the "neatly" part was really out of character). Plus, everything from all his drawers and closet was neatly folded and on his bed also. He said we had to go because the people who owned this house were coming and wanted to move back in. Since we had lived in the California house for 35 years and had just built this one, it was easy to see his confusion. It was another stab in my heart. Did I do the right thing? It's so hard to make all the decisions all by yourself. My love for him was so deep, I wanted to shelter and protect him as well as care for him. But one thing was sure—it was a done deal. We made room for him to lie down, and I snuggled with him until he went to sleep.

This is just one example of how it is so very difficult when the AD patient is your spouse. Had it been my parent, chances are good I'd have a spouse to consult on making the hard decisions. When incidents like this arose, I'd still have my spouse to provide validity that we made the right move. I'd have someone to hold and someone to hold me and provide comfort.

Our home sits on the first dune, which means the path leading to the surf takes about two minutes to walk. Our ocean home is in northern Washington. The water is cold and the wave action is treacherous, but it's beautiful to watch. We both loved to walk on the beach and see what had been churned up for us to find. I like the ordinary beach-combing items—shells, unusual driftwood shapes. Since Yogi had been a scuba instructor at a university, his interest was much more scientific. He would wander along the shoreline with our border collie, Zeke, with me close by. But sometimes I needed to do some housework—ugh! I would ask him to wait for me. That request would not always be remembered and I would frantically look all around outside the house, then race down the path to find him. With the ocean being so loud, it is impossible to hear from any distance. My running shoes went into action as I hustled to catch up with him, Zeke beside him.

One day during the cold, winter month of December this scenario was repeated, but I could not find him! I called the park rangers for help—I don't like to drive on the beach. When the rangers arrived, I gave them his photo. They went on their way, driving up and down the beach searching for him. Time passed into the evening and darkness fell, bringing a bitter chill. I worried about Zeke and Yogi being alone on the beach. If he was too tired he would sit with Zeke to keep each other a little warmer. I called my friend to help me cope with the situation. She in turn called our pastor. In a small town such as Westport, everyone participated in searches. There must have been eight vehicles— SUVs, jeeps, pickups—on the beach searching for Yogi and Zeke. Scores of prayers were being repeated. The park rangers called in the Coast Guard helicopter to expand the search with their spotlight. They would be able to survey the dunes as well as the shore. After hours of panic, tears, and prayers, we saw "the man and his dog" walking up our driveway. The paramedics checked him over and found him physically sound. All I could do was hug him and hug Zeke. Yogi really did not have any idea what was going on. He thought all those people came to visit and that we were having a great party.

Yogi loved people and was always ready for a party. After everyone left, I asked him where he had been. I wasn't expecting much of an answer, but it's a question you just have to ask. I also asked how he got home and wasn't he cold? All he said was "Zeke took me." Since that incident, I observed Zeke staying right by him whenever he went outside and saw that Zeke would bring him home if he wandered too far away. Sometimes Zeke had to come get me. Zeke would do so by barking at the deck door until I came to follow him. We always ended up right where Zeke had left his ward. What a dog.

Some things, actually all things, were challenging to wrap my head around. The task of remembering that he would forget moments after the situation occurred. Yogi liked to run the weed eater in the dune grass and would do so whether it was green or dry. On one occasion he cut down some very green grass and piled it into the fire pit. He proceeded to light match after match after match, rapidly emptying the box with nothing to show for it but black volumes of smoke. Our son Greg told him he could not light it. It was too green. "It would take a nuclear bomb to get it started." As we watched him try and fail over and over, it dawned on us that he would forget the match he had just tried, so of course, he would light another one, or in his case, the first one. It's still difficult to grasp his lapse of memory, but I firmly believed it was part of his life now. It really didn't matter to him if I knew this or didn't, but it helped me decipher a small part of the maze.

The wanderings were beginning to be a concern, especially when I would be gone all those days substituting. An arrangement was made for a caregiver to come to our home to stay with him until I returned. This was a great solution for this stage. Fred's memory was declining noticeably by the day. One evening a friend, Jim, brought over forty live crabs to cook, clean, eat, and freeze. Fred and Jim sat outside with the crab cooker, chatting, smoking cigars, drinking beer, and boiling crab. It was getting rather late. The crabs were placed into garbage bags in the garage fridge until morning when we would clean them. Morning found Yogi and me at a crab station. I had set up buckets for the backs, water for rinsing, and bags for storing them. After we had twenty of them cleaned. I put a full bag in the garage fridge and began the next twenty. When they were finished and in the bag, I told Fred to put the bag in the fridge while I went into the laundry room (about 20 feet away) to wash up. Big mistake! When I came back out, the crabs were not at the station. Had he in fact put the bag of crab in the garage fridge? Under the circumstances, I felt the need to check. Upon checking the fridge, I only found the first bag of twenty. I knew asking Fred would be futile, but I had to try. He replied, "What crab?" I proceeded to search for them—in the garage, in all the coolers, the trunk of the car, under the deck, in the nearby dunes—no crabs or bag! Thinking they would eventually begin to stink, or seagulls would start flocking around them, I gave up the search. We cleaned up the station and called it a day. No stench, no seagull flocks, no sign of the crabs ever presented itself. To this day, I have no idea what he did with them.

Holidays were bittersweet, and a major adjustment. I love

them—the decorating, the food, the family—everything except, I have to admit, when they're over. Not the taking down of decorations, the leftover food, and saying good-bye to family. I did the "Family Christmas Event" every year, going all-out in the decorating part. It was almost frantic. One year I had five real trees, even one in the bathroom. It's funny when the inside is hurting, I felt the need sparkle up the outside. Yogi seemed to like all the activities, for the moment. One Thanksgiving after he had moved into David's home, we planned a special excursion to the local hotel in Tokeland for a turkey-day dinner. The hotel is a famous old-style facility, with antiques in every room. It was close to home. Greg and all three of his kids, Kyle, Kellie, and Katie, who had always been special to Fred, came up from California. They were all grown up, but Yogi still remembered them, I think. I had decided to go to the hotel instead of having dinner at David's because chaos agitated Yogi, and all the movement, TV noise, and people coming in and out might be too much for him. It definitely would be for me. It was a great time. It was a memory for us and at the same time, a painful acceptance of the inevitable. Holidays would never be the same.

There *are* some pluses in this merry-go-round. No reruns on TV; each episode is brand new. No leftovers; each dish was never served before. No sorrow; no one has died—all are still living, even his parents and mine. Everything is brand-new no matter how many times it's been told, tasted, felt, or seen. Some patients, so I've been told or read about, get violent. In that regard I was lucky. Yogi's "lover attitude" stayed with him. He was a sweet, caring, compassionate man and remained so. It made him easier to care for, but also made me sadder that I couldn't "fix" it. The human part of me does not want to write this part, but it would not be true if I did not, and it might help someone. I would get extremely impatient and yell at him when he would do something that was not correct—and that was just about everything, all the time. I *knew* he could not help it, but I wanted him to so desperately. Plus, he still did not look any different. Then the guilt would set in. Believe it or not, I wanted to blame him for that too. The reality of Alzheimer's was settling into my heart and soul.

Our two boys—not boys, men in their forties—found it very difficult. Our oldest son, Greg, would bravely take him for day fishing trips, and even weekend ones. Yogi would grumble and complain all the way until he got there. Then of course, he was the *only* one who knew how to fish. Some things were slow to change. Those memories left Yogi as soon as he returned home, but they would stay with Greg for a lifetime. Yogi developed fears that he had not shown before. One day he was getting ready to go with David for the night. He got to the porch and the three steps leading to the driveway. He started shaking and was very fearful. He would stand on the top step and try to step down but just couldn't. Greg was on one side, I was on the other, and David was in front of him trying to coax him down. He just stood there and shook with fear, until Greg picked him up like a baby and carried him to the van. That picture of our son carrying his dad in his arms shattered me. Every one of these milestones hit me square in my gut, leaving a large, hurting hole in my heart. I had read where spatial awareness was sometimes greatly altered in AD patients. His standing on the steps was equivalent to you and me standing at the edge of the Grand Canyon and being told, "Take a step!"

Greg loved to do the things he always had done with his dad. Things like fishing. We figured a fishing trip would be good for all. As for me, I would be alone for a while. This would be Dad and son's time together. Oops, there's that word again—together—just not there anymore. They launched the boat, called *Nightmare*— which could have been an omen—into the Chehalis River and they got through the day. But when it came time to take the boat out, problems arose. Greg asked his dad to hold the rope while he got the boat trailer. Dad did it dutifully, actually quite proud of himself. When Greg returned, he found Dad holding the rope like he was asked to do—while watching the boat sink. He asked his son, "Is it supposed to do that?" Before Alzheimer's he would have known the plug was out and needed to be put back in, but not now. He just stood there and watched while Greg scrambled to re-plug it. Greg, like all of us, was frustrated that his dad could not do those things he had taught Greg to do when he was a boy. Roles definitely switched.

We lived on a beach that you can drive on, but only certain times of the year. Greg drove his brother's Durango SUV down on the beach with his dad one rainy, foggy winter day. Not seeing because of the fog or maybe just not heeding the sign listing restrictive dates, they were stopped by a park ranger. The ranger spotted the open beer can Yogi had and told him he'd have to dump it out. Wrong move by the ranger. That was *not* going to happen. Yogi looked at him, then at his son, then at the can of beer, in that sequence, about three times. He took a long look at the ranger and gave him "the hand message" of exactly how he felt, rolled up the window, and contently drank his beer. The ranger was ready to arrest him for defiance until Greg explained Yogi's situation to him. The park ranger was very gracious about it and just asked to see the registration of the vehicle. The vehicle belonged to Bob, who was deployed in Iraq, and the registration was in his name. The ranger went to look it up because they could not find it in the pickup. He returned to say there was no Durango registered in the name of Siler. Greg rightly figured out it was probably registered in his brother's wife's maiden name, a name Greg could not remember. The officer was becoming suspicious when all of a sudden, Dad piped up with "Ramento." That was her maiden name. How he remembered that obscure bit of information defies logic.

Alzheimer's has no logic.

We bought a ski boat back when I started teaching decades

earlier. This boat gave Dad and sons many memories of water skiing and salmon fishing. Yogi must have had great pictures in his mind of times in that boat, because he looked for that boat every time he got in the car when we were in Westport. We kept telling him we sold it 25 years ago, but he would not—or could not—accept that. Once when Greg told him we sold it, he asked, "Where's the money?" Some things remained important to him, like money. Greg and Yogi were returning to Eureka, California, and stopped at a Crescent City casino along the way. Not knowing how to play the slots he just started pushing buttons. Greg tried to stop him but was too late. He had pushed the "max bet" button and the brightly glowing machine responded. Yogi won! He squirreled the $1,800 away and did not share a cent. There were times when he was childlike.

Well, it was that time. The two Davids would care for Yogi in their foster home as caregivers. Previously, David had been coming to our home to stay with Yogi while I substituted at the local elementary school. It was no longer safe to leave him alone. The possibility of him falling and being unable to get up was becoming more and more plausible. Bathroom and kitchen accidents, fire hazards from his cigar smoking, as well as wandering off and becoming lost—the thought was frightening. Having a full-time caregiver had become a necessity for peace of mind.

In our forties, Yogi had good foresight into our future when he decided to purchase long-term health insurance. David's pay was covered, and he was only 15 miles away. David would come to our home when I was called into the school, which was quite often. Thus, Yogi became used to having him around. I'm not sure what he "actually" thought when David would drop by, spend the day, and leave when I returned. I felt it transitioned from entertaining a guest to being comfortable living with a guest. Either way, he never mentioned it to me.

Yogi referred to where he was staying as "home" and settled

in quite comfortably. I put pictures and other things in his room, hung his clothes in the closet, and visited with him as often as I could. It was extremely difficult for me to visit with him there. I had so many emotions about it. I sorely missed Yogi, but not *this* Yogi—the one who would fall and I could not get him up; the one who would wander off and I could not find him; the one I had to treat and care for like I did for our toddlers. The tears I shed on the ride back home were for both of us. I had always leaned on and depended on him and now it was reversed. I felt we were both lost, but I had to find the paths we needed to travel. I do not and did not know if they were right or wrong, best or worst, but they were all I knew or could gather from other sources.

While Yogi was in "the home," I rented a transporter to bring him out to our house for visits. By this time he was in a wheelchair and had to be fed. He seemed to like the visits, but he liked leaving too. Being in "the home" necessitated trips to the emergency room quite often. By law, they had to take residents in whenever their temperature or blood pressure became elevated or their breathing became labored. Yogi was no exception. The first time David called and told me the ambulance was taking him to ER, my heart stopped. I sped over to beat the ambulance. However, after the umpteenth time it happened, I obeyed the speed limits. One time we were in the emergency room, and the catheter was inserted, which usually left me with bruised hands as he was petrified of it. His nurse was filling out her chart. She was a nice looking, middle-aged lady, nothing to make you look twice— except for Yogi. He kept looking and looking at her, then finally motioned her over to his bedside. He seriously and politely asked her: "Have you ever worked in a whorehouse?" We all gasped, turned red, then howled! I should have asked him, "Why? Does she look familiar?" Hindsight. Yogi had been, and apparently still was, a flirt—and a successful one.

When he got to "the home" he was "king"—being the only

male among five female residents. He would flatter each and every one of them. There was one in particular who "fit." Sadly, I'm very jealous. But I tried to ignore this situation and attribute it where it belonged—Alzheimer's. They ate together and I came to realize the attraction. It was for food. She did not like to eat, so she'd put a piece here and a piece there on Yogi's plate, which he had no problem with. But they say jealousy is a green-eyed monster and my eyes are green. When she passed on, it did not even register with him. That was another blessing; he did not remember the deaths of anyone.

As I sat with Yogi and flipped through one of our photo albums I remembered things he used to do that used to irritate me. He would stay out with "the guys" longer than he should have and drink more than he ought. One time when this occurred he called me to come and get him. We had two toddlers asleep who I had to bundle into the car—a VW bug—not an easy task. I'd drive and pick him up, fuming. He was happy because he was a happy drunk. I drove home, got my babies out, went up the stairs and back into bed. I looked out the window at the car where I had left Yogi, as he did not follow me up the flight of stairs. There he was … half-in, half-out of the passenger side, passed out on the lawn. Looking at it now I had two options, go get him or leave him. However, at that time I felt I only had one option. I was so angry at him that I turned out the light and went to bed.

I'd give anything to have problems like that again. We had a great marriage. Even great marriages have bumps and ours was certainly no different. This Alzheimer's was not a bump, it was a mountain. I guess even mountains need to be crossed. It's funny how the memories of the past, at least some of the memories, just will not leave the present. It was so difficult to go and visit him. I usually cried all the way home. I worried, what will I find? Does it matter? There are personal questions that only the people involved can address. I wrestled with a new set every week.

Questions like, Am I doing all I can? What is the best thing to do? I even questioned if I should have told him he had Alzheimer's at the diagnosis. Did I take away his right to decide? There were plenty of things we tried. We would look at old photos, our children, play his favorite music.

I had exhausted the medical field for answers, suggestions, medical alternatives, and advice. He had monthly visits with neurologists and his family doctor. They prescribed Aricept and Namenda to slow down the progress until I came to the point where I felt it was not right to keep him in the state he was in instead of just letting go. There are all the personal decisions included to tell only our story. I had decorated his room with memories. I added pictures of places and people on the walls and on dresser tops, until they became a hazard. He was losing his balance and would fall against them, against the dressers, the walls, knocking off and knocking down the pictures, bruising or cutting himself. He began to fall out of bed. We tried putting a long body pillow under the side sheet. When that stopped working, we cleared out the night stand, which he would hit when he fell and put a thick section of foam rubber covered with a sheet on the floor beside and under his bed. Voila! Soft landing. I tried very hard to keep him comfortable and as "well" as I knew how.

He showed signs of cataracts, so we (David and I and the transport guy, who became a very good friend) took him to an ophthalmologist. It was like the "Keystone Kops" to examine him, because he did not quite get what he was supposed to do, where to place his head, how long to keep it there, and so on. He was surrounded by medical people and I could not get to him. I finally crawled on the floor between their legs and reached for his hand.

Their test was completed and he was scheduled for the removal of one cataract. Yogi was required to sleep for the procedure. I waited and waited, becoming worried, then scared, then alarmed after four hours had elapsed. The procedure usually took

30 minutes. The doctor finally came out—looking very haggard—to tell me, "That was the cataract from hell." He literally had to "dig" it out. I believe he submitted the operating procedure to the American Medical Association. After all that, he said Yogi should be able to see much more clearly out of that eye. He did not plan on operating on the other eye because of the severity of the eye and Yogi's rapidly declining condition. I needed to be sure he could see as they could not "test" him the regular way.

One afternoon I was visiting and sitting next to him on the couch. I was flipping through a catalogue he liked to look at also. I came upon a page advertising bras and Yogi sat up straighter, took the catalogue, and looked. Yes, I knew he could see again. Not long after that, I got a call from David telling me to come quickly, as Yogi's breathing was not good. Once again, I sped to "the home" to find the paramedics preparing to load him onto a gurney. He was in bed. I crawled across to where he was and kissed him on the cheek. He looked at me and smiled. I have put many different meanings into that smile in the years following. My favorite one is that, at that moment we were back in the student union building at the University of Oregon. They put Yogi in a room to monitor him with my instructions of DNR, only to give him hydration and morphine. As much as I wanted him back, the reality of him coming back in his current state was not what I wanted or what I knew he would want. Our sons arrived. Greg had been with me, and Bob came from Gig Harbor, Washington. When Bob walked through the hospital door and saw his dad, he literally fell onto his knees. Yogi did not resemble the "Yogi" we knew and loved. He died the next day with me, my sister, and our sons around him.

I had him cremated and held onto his ashes. Why? I did not know, but God did. I was not going to have a service, as we had moved from the place where all of our former friends lived. I just sat on the couch and breathed. Then, when the phone calls came in from former players, coaches, buddies, and friends asking when his memorial would be, I began to think they needed closure even if I did not. Yogi had been such a larger than life presence it was difficult for them to grasp him not being here any longer. I planned to have a celebration of his life six months after his death. I asked a dear church friend to take our family out on his boat to spread Yogi's ashes in the ocean he loved so much. His family—my sister and I, Yogi's sons and grandkids—and Mike (a special friend) each took a small part of Yogi, Dad, Grandpa and coach in a small bottle and poured it into the ocean, along with a U of O wreath of yellow mums floating on top. After a few words, we returned to our home for food and many stories. It was a great tribute to a fantastic guy.

Time teaches one to cherish the moment, however brief it may be. The tendency to compare what he/we used to be can rip a person apart. Instead, I tried to look forward to a smile, to holding his hand, those moments that happen one day that he would forget the next. But I won't. I need and needed those special moments. Each step is worse than the last one but not as bad as the next. Cherish what you have, when you have it. The latest news of the numerous research projects to prevent, cure, arrest Alzheimer's will eat away at your soul. The "if only" haunted and still haunts me. If only I had … What if … Did I check … and so on. At the time, I felt I had left no stone unturned. But I realized I may not know all the stones. I took Yogi to neurology specialists in Seattle and investigated any and all Alzheimer trial studies at the University of Washington Medical School. The specialists performed an MRI and reported no tumors, bleeding, or growths. The trial groups would not include Yogi because he smoked cigars. I tried Aricept, then Namenda, then Aricept with Namenda, seeing very little difference. We continued seeing the neurologist once a month for four years … just in case? Until I arrived at the final stage … acceptance. Elisabeth Kubler-Ross's stages of grieving became a description of my emotional existence. I went from denial to trying to "fix" it, to debilitating self-pity, to lost and forlorn, and finally I accepted the inevitable. When this became my reality, I canceled the neurologist and stopped the medications that were supposed to "slow down" the progression of the disease. I did not want it to slow down. I did not want to keep it where it was because it was at the worst possible place to be. I just wanted to get on with it. It took ten years for me to reach this feeling. I rested in my decision and hated myself at the time. Looking back on it, I do not feel I should have done it any differently.

We all must listen to and follow our own hearts, no one else's. It's a very private journey, and one you'll need to do all by yourself.

DEDICATED TO:
ARDITH "PENNY" MARDELLE NORQUIST ALLEN
1933–2013 (79 YEARS OLD)

Ardith was born in International Falls, Minnesota, in December 1933. The Falls was called the ice box of the nation, with recorded temperatures exceeding 50 below zero, not counting the wind chill factor. She enjoyed the early days of her youth playing with cousins on Grandpa's farm. In her early teens the family moved to Minneapolis, where she enjoyed ice skating on the numerous outdoor rinks, lakes, and ponds in the city. She attended Sunday School at a Baptist church. With her father in heavy construction and road building, they criss-crossed the country from Minnesota to California, back to Minnesota, then to Oregon. Back again to Minnesota again before settling in Sweet Home, Oregon, a booming logging town of 1,500 people.

In her freshman year of high school, her friends "changed" her name to Penny because of her red hair. She achieved above average grades in all her studies, but excelled in bookkeeping, shorthand, and typing, in which she was tops in her class. Penny wrote a gossip column for the school paper that earned her a journalism scholarship at the University of Oregon. One of the more popular girls in school, Penny participated in activities that included serving as a class officer, majorette, rally girl, and a reporter for the school paper. She was selected as a May Day

Princess, the Sweetheart's Ball Queen, and became a princess for the Albany Timber Carnival, a county and state event.

After graduation from high school, Penny worked at the local bank until the GM auto dealership offered her the position of bookkeeper and receptionist. She won awards for excellent bookkeeping from General Motors Accounting Corporation. In June of 1952, she married D. Matt Allen, a classmate. She studied and was confirmed into the Lutheran religion. Six months later, Matt was drafted into the Korean War. After his basic training, Penny joined him in California. After he completed Signal Corps training, she traveled with him to his next duty station—Camp Gordon, Georgia. In Augusta, Penny began working as a medical stenographer for a medical research doctor from New York with an office and laboratory in Augusta. She would accompany the doctor to the Milledgeville State Hospital for Women. His research perfected the Pap test for women.

After the birth of their first daughter, her husband's company became support staff to the first atomic cannon firing exercises in the Armed Forces at Fort Bragg, North Carolina. Mother and one-month-old daughter flew back to Oregon. While flying over the snow-covered Rockies, the pilot came back to her seat, giving instructions on how to protect her baby in a forced—or crashed—landing on a glacier. Ice was building up on the wings and the plane could not hold altitude. She kept reciting the Lord's Prayer—and He answered. Ice began breaking off the wings as the Lockheed "Super Connie" weaved among the mountain tops.

Returning to Georgia, Penny recalled their introduction to the hostile, segregated South ... bombing of city buses, murders and rapes in their neighborhood. They longed to be back home in their rough 'n' tough logging town in Oregon. Their trip back to Oregon was a test of their faith. Matt drove all night from Austin, Texas. Wrong decision. A blinding snowstorm kept them on high alert until dawn. "Thank you Lord for our new Chevy hard-top."

The heater kept them from freezing and the defrosters kept ice from building up on the windshield. He drove with the right tire at the edge of the pavement. It was a "white out"—they could not see beyond the hood ornament. Back on the West Coast, they again enjoyed great coffee (they drank chicory in the South) and no grits! Matt returned to work with his old crew of logging engineers. Penny took a position as a full charge bookkeeper at a plywood mill. Try handling twice-a-month payroll for 250 workers and keeping the "rolling" plywood inventory of railroad box cars throughout the nation—without a computer. She did have an assistant, plus 10-key adding machines and manual typewriters. One year between jobs, she filled in for a high school classmate who took a much deserved two-week vacation. Penny became the office manager for Timber Service in Sweet Home. They managed the Hill family timber holdings (over 200 sections in the Willamette National Forest). The Hill family also owned 3M and the Great Northern Railroad. Eventually, Penny went back to her position as office manager and accountant at the GM auto dealership.

In September of 1955, Matt enrolled at Oregon State College (now University) to study engineering. His schoolmate, who was just out of the Navy, joined him at OSC as a pre-med student. They commuted 75 miles a day for four years. During those four years, Penny's parents divorced, drawing her into their feud. She was near a nervous breakdown. Her mother was a heavy drinker of bourbon. Matt took a position in Portland, and once more they were away from the influence of her mother.

Penny was a "stay at home mom" until their second daughter was four. She took a position with a major department store in Portland. This was her love—sales. Her position (which was created for her by the manager) was envied by other sales clerks. In women's fashions, she could sell merchandise in any department. If a gentleman wished to purchase a sweater for his wife or girlfriend, Penny would also sell him a skirt, slacks, blouse, etc.

Of course, with her great personality, model's figure, and dark red hair she excelled in the department. They bought their first home—in Southeast Portland. On their street they had the four top glamour queens in the neighborhood—two platinum blondes, a brunette, and a redhead. They enjoyed the nightlife in Portland's jazz scene, and loved swing dancing. Penny was a great ballroom dancer; she made Matt look good. Two clubs in Portland played her "theme song" whenever they stepped onto the dance floor: "Pennies From Heaven."

Matt had a heart attack at the age of 37. A warning. He lost his job as a sales engineer for a foundry. He was out of work, and no firm would hire him with a heart attack on his record. Penny went back to work for an MD as his bookkeeper and eventually his office manager. Matt started his own business as a manufacturer's representative, and it took a couple years to build up his income. In the meantime, they had a daughter in college (on scholarships) and one in middle school.

Penny phased the doctor into retirement and he died a year later. As a father figure, his passing brought another difficult time in her life. Within a couple weeks, she was offered the position of office manager for another doctor. This doctor compromised her integrity. He had financial problems with banks and the IRS. Penny moved on to another doctor, an OB/GYN, a gifted lady. Penny finally found her passion. She was with this doctor until they both retired. Her family held an intervention that curtailed her drinking for two months. She never neglected her family, and her drinking never affected her work. She was an impeccable, full-charge bookkeeper—without the help of a computer.

After being diagnosed with AD she continued drinking wine until she stopped when Matt convinced her that the alcohol was not allowing her medications and supplements to be effective and help her. Did the alcohol consumption contribute to Alzheimer's? It is considered a co-factor. It surely did not improve her brain's function.

CHAPTER 1

MOTHER–MID-1980s–
EARLY DIAGNOSIS

Fifteen years after my father's death, my mom was secure with enough money to provide for her into the future plus a modest home left to her by her stepfather. As her financial adviser, my worries were over—I thought. We noticed signs of senility, or could it be Alzheimer's disease? At that time, mid-1980s, medical authorities claimed the only way to determine if a person had Alzheimer's was after death, through an autopsy. I scheduled Mom for an appointment with her MD. His observation was comforting but unusual.

"Your mother's getting a little senile—nothing to be concerned about."

After that statement he diverted into a conversation about his mother, who was senile. Apparently, the doctor was in denial about his mother's mental condition. I scheduled an appointment for Mom with my MD. After a brief examination and discussion, my doctor went into the same rationalization. The same thing happened with a third MD. This was becoming quite interesting.

They all had a mother experiencing the same problems. However, in all three examples the doctors themselves were in denial.

With my wife being the office manager of a small medical clinic and our daughter a nurse, I had access to numerous medical publications. I noticed an article mentioning a local medical center being awarded a grant from the federal government to conduct a study on memory loss—Alzheimer's disease. I contacted the group and asked if my mother could qualify as a patient in their study. They replied with great enthusiasm, and we scheduled an appointment. As I was filling out the required paperwork, I noticed a line that asked for the name of her insurance company. She was on Medicare, plus she had a private policy. When I asked questions, they advised me their fee for the test was $2,500, but not to worry, it would be covered by Medicare and the insurance company. Was this a rip-off? A scam? The medical center received a multimillion dollar grant and they're billing the patients? Is that double billing?

Our family made the diagnosis. We reviewed Mom's daily routine and financial matters:

A. I had power of attorney and was listed as an additional signature on her bank accounts.

B. I reviewed her check stubs. She would send checks to numerous evangelists.

They sent a letter asking for money, usually, weekly. She paid for "additional" police protection, although she was the only one in the neighborhood who did, being the oldest. When I asked younger families in the neighborhood, they had not been asked to pay for additional police protection. How interesting. Even the ones you expect to protect your interests are reaching into your pockets. A local septic tank service talked Mom into having her septic tank pumped out. Strange. Her home had been on the city sewer line for several years. I got her money back. I wonder if these jokers pass old widows' names around—"Hey, old lady Smith is senile and can't remember much. I'll bet you can con her out of a new roof job."

C. Her "new church" (she left the Lutheran church where she had been a member since childhood) held a "financial analysis" meeting for their older members. Somehow, they found out how much money she had in her numerous bank accounts, her mutual funds, and the value of her property within a few thousand dollars. There was no way that she knew. But her church somehow "received" the information. When I asked who appraised her property, she said it was Brother Ray from her church. I visited her bank and spoke with the manager. When I suggested that someone in his bank might be giving out confidential information, he insisted it was none of his people. At that moment, a young teller excused herself while glancing at me. Her face was red with guilt. I suggested that he ask the young teller who was scurrying to their break room. I closed out Mom's accounts in that bank. I never inquired about the mutual fund group, but I had my suspicions.

D. To improve her cash situation I had her property divided to increase the value and a possible sale. When I visited the county for permits and planning, their staff seemed to be very incompetent or extremely vindictive. Finally, I found someone who went through the records to show that a real estate developer had put a claim on Mom's property. When her stepfather died and the property was willed to Mom, some good ol' boy in the neighborhood tried to pull a fast one. The lady at the county said sometimes they get away with it. But this time he could not produce a valid bill of sale. The division of the property provided additional cash to invest.

E. Her attorney called one afternoon. Mom and four people from her new church were in his office. He said they were there to change her will. Shocked, I rushed down to his office. When I asked her what she was doing, she said she was changing her will to give all her money to the church. She seemed upset with my sister and me. It was as if she had been the victim of brain-washing. Mom went into a private room with her attorney, at his request. When they came out he advised the church group and me that Mrs. Allen had no intention of changing her will. I never said a word to her church friends, but they expressed bitterness toward me for "stealing the church money."

F. One evening Mom called saying she was selling her home, cashing in her mutual funds, etc., and converting every asset to gold. When I asked why, she said the world was coming to an end. Again, her church was holding their brainwashing sessions with the older members. I talked her out of the idea.

G. Life insurance salesmen became a thorn in my side. They would try to sell her a policy. Luckily, she would call me for advice. I kept reminding her that she had adequate insurance. I would talk with the salesmen and tell them she was well covered. Two salesmen were very persistent. They tried to sell her a policy with an upfront premium. One wanted $2,500 and the other wanted $3,000. When I told them we were not interested, they kept coming back, hoping to find her alone. I thought I had heard the last of them. I received two phone calls from her bank. They said she was trying to withdraw cash ($2,500 and $3,000). I had the bank manager put the salesman on the phone.

"Do you understand *no*? You leave my mother alone or I'll file a lawsuit against you and your firm for harassment." It seems like there's always some culprit out there trying to scam old widows who have a bank account. I had the bank remove Mom's name from her accounts and I became her guardian.

It was obvious. Mom was having problems living by herself. To the unscrupulous in our society, she was a pigeon. Frequently, she would call in a panic. It was 95 degrees in her home (in January) and she could not turn down the thermostat. Thinking it might be a faulty switch, I drove out to her home only to find that she had *forgotten* how to set the thermostat. On another occasion, when I went out to her home to do some work, I noticed an old coat hanging on a hook behind the kitchen door. The sleeve material had "burn rings" from being on the element on her electric range when the burner was on low. She could have caused a fire. Her memory was not too bad, but her logic and judgment were gone.

She drove into a neighbor's driveway, four houses down, thinking it was our home. She could not tell where she was or how to get to our home. I had her doctor request a driver's license exam rather than tell her she couldn't drive. She flunked the exam at the Department of Motor Vehicles.

It's better to have the doctor request a driver's license exam than a family member to get involved. I convinced Mom that it was in her best interests. "You may get a sore arm or a dented fender, but what if you hurt a child … maybe broke their leg or arm?"

We knew she had to leave her home or hire a live-in caregiver—but who could we trust? One way to see if loved ones require personal help is to review their refrigerator. Mom had six containers of ice cream and over a dozen cartons of eggs, some dating back nearly a year. There were no fresh vegetables. She did have a few apples, oranges, and bananas. Most of her food was canned goods, which required turning on the burner of her range. She was taking a few supplements—brewer's yeast, rose hips, and a multi-vitamin.

Years after her death, while perusing her health books, authored by Paavo Airola, PhD, ND, I came across pages where the term "pernicious anemia" was marked. In checking her old medical files, I found that she had been diagnosed with pernicious anemia. It is a vitamin B_{12} deficiency where the stomach does not produce an enzyme, thus vitamin B_{12} cannot be absorbed and utilized. The vitamin is required for building red blood cells and proper neurological function. After her doctor realized she had AD, she received weekly injections of vitamin B_{12}. Was it too late?

It's not easy relocating an older person out of their home, especially not with Mom and her two cats. My family had good intentions, but you just can't drag someone from their front porch, getting slivers under their fingernails. It wasn't quite *that* bad, but I'm sure you get my point. After three conversations with doctors, we finally received good, logical advice. The counselor at Kaiser Permanente suggested we take Mom to a relative for a two-week change of environment. My aunt, Mom's sister-in-law, agreed to have Mom spend the time with her. She lived alone on a farm with family and friends close by. A granddaughter lived in a modular home on her property. After one week, my aunt called in desperation. Mom was too much to handle. She was pacing the floor, repeatedly asking questions, getting into things, getting up at night and wandering, etc. But that one week allowed us time to move Mom's bedroom set and clothes into our daughter's home.

Our daughter Debbie, a nurse, agreed to care of Grandma. This was not an easy decision for her and her husband, Bob. Their daughter was born with spina bifida, a birth defect. Our daughter and her husband now cared for two people with special medical and health needs. Mom lived with our daughter's family, next door to our home, for more than three years. During that period our daughter gave birth to twin girls. Taking care of everyone became more than a full-time job. We hired a young woman to help her. By now, Mom was near the point of needing to be placed in an adult foster home.

Our daughter called one night near midnight, almost crying,

"Dad, we need you." I hurried over to their home to find Mom in the bath tub. While she was on the toilet, she had pooped, and with her hands smeared the matter on the walls and herself (care-givers at the AD facilities call this "painting"). Bob was tending to their older daughter who had problems and Debbie was com-forting the twins. I gave Mom a bath, dressed her, and finally got her back in bed. To allow Debbie and Bob to catch their breath, we temporarily placed Mom in an adult foster home for a couple weeks. We were also "testing the waters," so to speak, until we found a good permanent foster home. The owner of the foster home called the day I was to bring Mom back to Debbie's home.

"Your mother may tell you a story that I will explain. During the night a male resident wandered into your mother's room and tried to get in bed with her. I swear nothing happened." When I arrived, Mom was all smiles with her overnight case ready to come home. But before we left, she took me to the room of the "wandering Don Juan" and introduced me to her new friend, an Italian gentleman in his nineties. By the time we arrived home at Debbie's, the 90-year-old gent became a 70-year-old Italian Don Juan. After Mom made a few phone calls to her friends (with Debbie monitoring), the "wandering Don Juan" had become a 30-year-old man from Mexico who was attracted to her.

There were times when Mom became somewhat entertaining; you must have a proper attitude to cope with these issues. Debbie said Mom would ask her, "When is that lady coming to pick up her kids?" Mom could not understand why Debbie's children were in her (Mom's) home.

Bob was startled one night when Grandma got out of bed and wandered. They left lights on in the hallway in the event Grandma got up to use the bathroom. She could not find her bed-room, but eventually, she made it to Debbie and Bob's bedroom. Grandma pulled back the covers and slid her cold, bony fingers across Bob's stomach and touched his rig! That brought him out of a sound sleep.

She would "play" with her dentures, removing the lower plate and replacing it with one side sticking outside her mouth. It was frightening to the children. They thought she was trying to scare them.

We found an ideal foster home for Mom. The caregivers would call me when Mom asked for me in between my visits. During the first few months, she kept asking me when she would be going home. It took her four years to lose memory of me. First, it was recognition of my face. Finally, it was my voice. She could not detect that I was her son by my voice. When I visited, she would be walking around the home or sitting at the table with other residents. She was the only one with AD. Mom died in January of 1993, 10 years after she displayed moderate signs of Alzheimer's disease.

TAKE ACTION

If you have an elderly relative or dear friend living alone, without anyone to care for them, take the necessary steps to ensure that they are receiving proper nutrition and care. Assist them if you think there is a need by discussing durable powers of attorney for health care and financial matters and their will. Obtain from your doctor's office, or theirs, the forms (advance directive) for making health care decisions.

MAINTAIN CONTROL

A business colleague of mine encountered a sad experience of greed. Bill and his wife had cared for an elderly lady for years. They took her out to dinner and concerts. They became her only close friends. She had no relatives. Years before her death, she made out her will, leaving them her historic Victorian home with three floors of antiques. Her will stipulated they could never sell her home, but they could live in it until their death. At the time of their death (either one), the home would be sold along with the antiques, with the money going to a couple charities for children that she listed in the Portland area. When it was time for her to move to a nursing home (she revealed signs of Alzheimer's), they took care of all the arrangements and visited her a few times a week. When near death after an illness, she was transferred to a hospital. They continued their visits (but not 24/7), and within days she died. Bill and his wife presented their copy of her will to their attorney. Her will giving them her home and antiques was invalid.

Another will had taken precedence. It was dated after she entered the hospital, and was written by an attorney with no link to their friend.

The *new* attorney became the recipient of her estate. Where did this ambulance chaser come from? How could this possibly happen? How would he know about her? How would he know she was vulnerable and dying in a hospital? Unless someone in the hospital tipped him off, he had no way of knowing. Do they post elderly people with no relatives that enter hospitals on an attorney bulletin board? Bill and his wife appealed, but the judge denied the appeal, awarding the estate to the attorney. Was the judge in on the legal scam? The attorney sold the home and antiques through an estate sale without a dime going to the children's charities. I wonder if the proceeds were split three ways—the doctor, the lawyer, and the judge. Maybe just two.

CHAPTER 2

UNCLE CARL

During our fight to maintain control of the wealth Mom had accumulated, another estate problem surfaced in California. My wife's aunt Betty and uncle Carl were financially secure. Her aunt retired as an office manager from a utility district. Her uncle retired as an electrical engineer from Shell Oil. They had lived in a very nice home in the Bay Area. But since retirement they had moved to a city in Stanislaus County. With their stocks, bonds, savings, antiques, and real property, they had a net worth over $2 million. In that the couple had no children and my wife's uncle was an orphan, they had a joint will leaving everything to family, my wife being one of four named in their will. Her aunt's only brother had both general and real estate power of attorney. When her aunt died a couple years prior, the joint will revealed the distribution of their estate to Uncle Ben and the family members, upon the death of Uncle Carl. With his wife gone, Uncle Carl became lonely. He lived with his brother-in-law for a few months and they both visited friends in the Midwest. In his eighties, Uncle Carl was in need of a housekeeper, someone to help him around his large three-bedroom home. When his wife was alive, Uncle Carl did all the cooking. Friends from the Midwest suggested a young woman, in her early twenties, who would move to California to attend a Bible college in Uncle Carl's city. Kathy could stay with Uncle Carl and help with the house chores for her room and board.

With Uncle Ben having the power of attorney and the existence of the joint will there was no worry—after all, the young woman was a "born-again" Christian. The last thing that entered the minds of the family was the young Christian woman trying to steal from his estate. We received cards from Uncle Carl and Kathy when they were traveling in Arizona, California, Idaho, New Mexico, Minnesota, and Wisconsin. Uncle Carl's health was failing. Although we never knew he had heart problems, he was hospitalized from three heart attacks within a few months. In the spring of 1987, we received word that Uncle Carl had died from a heart attack. My wife and Uncle Ben drove down for the funeral and reading of the will. I stayed home to help with Mom, plus I had a manufacturing business with defense contracts to operate.

After the reading of the will, my wife called, extremely upset: "That little bitch Kathy got Uncle Carl's estate ... his home, all the furnishings, their antiques, his car, their stocks and bonds and bank accounts ... everything except a token amount of $1,000 to each of our family members. That little 'born-again' Christian cleaned us out."

Uncle Ben would contest the will. They tried to retain a local attorney, but could not locate an attorney who would take the case, when they discovered Kathy had retained one of the most unscrupulous attorneys in Stanislaus County. He was also a part-time preacher. Without Uncle Carl's knowledge, a *new* attorney wrote a *new* will, per Kathy's instructions which, according to California laws, superseded the original joint will. Apparently she had planned this for months. Uncle Ben called me to see if any of my attorney friends could suggest an attorney to take the case in Stan-islaus County. A law firm in Oakland was suggested. Uncle Ben and my wife drove home. The following week, Uncle Ben and I visited the law firm in Oakland and briefed them on the case. They reviewed their information on Kathy's attorney and the presiding judge. It was not good. The attorney was close to being disbarred, and the judge was questionable. It was destined to be a shootout between unethical attorneys from a small city and the big city attorneys that represented a major religious group in the Bay Area.

Kathy was not staying in Uncle Carl's home. We stayed in his home gathering information and evidence that Kathy forgot to remove. We talked with neighbors. I brought home a briefcase full of receipts, canceled checks, and other incriminating evidence. Kathy's attorney gave us an inventory of items that Kathy would keep and we could have the rest—junk. They missed many "family collectible" items that were in the attic that Uncle Carl forgot. No doubt Uncle Carl was in the middle stage of Alzheimer's disease, although, to our knowledge, he was never diagnosed. In those days (mid-1980s) AD was considered senility. In the evenings, after going through all of Uncle Carl's files, I listed all the purchases, contracts and unusual canceled checks, credit card receipts, etc.

1. He paid $9,000 for worthless stock from his neighbor.

2. His church borrowed $25,000. "Loan" was written on the check.

3. His friend and fishing partner, a Cadillac salesman, sold him a new Oldsmobile—over sticker price—and allowed him a mere $1,500 for his two-year-old Cadillac El Dorado that had 8,000 miles on the odometer. Nice way to treat an old fishing buddy.

4. His neighbor, a nurse, claimed Kathy was giving him too much heart medication.

5. The bank allowed Kathy to remove bonds, stocks, cash, etc., from safety deposit box.

6. Kathy was forging Aunt Betty's name on credit cards months after her death.

7. Kathy was depositing checks from Uncle Carl to her bank account in Wisconsin. The largest one was for $8,000, and was marked "loan."

8. The bank refused to produce records of Uncle Carl's account. Later, they said they were lost. Out of 2,000 accounts, Uncle Carl's were the only ones lost. The bank was found in contempt of court.

9. Kathy's friend in Wisconsin called to say she would be a witness against Kathy, claiming Kathy said she was after the old man's money. Another person who knew this "friend" said she was also a "born again" Christian, and attended Kathy's church in Wisconsin. She was also the director of a national girls' foundation. She flew out in her father's corporate jet, but once on the witness stand, her testimony supported Kathy. Uncle Ben's attorneys did not use this "sweet, ethical, born again Christian" as a witness.

10. I tallied what Uncle Carl and Aunt Betty spent a year for daily living expenses. Then I tallied what Uncle Carl and Kathy had been spending in a 12-month period, not including trips. It was three times as much, not including checks Kathy made out to herself. If Uncle Carl wrote her a check, he noted "loan." If she wrote checks, she forged his name and the bank cashed them.

Many people in this city were fleecing Uncle Carl—the Cadillac salesman, his preacher, his neighbor, the bank, and who knows how many others. Uncle Ben and I drove home with a few items of interest to the family. I was sure that if Kathy got everything she would have an estate sale and dispose of all the family treasures from Aunt Betty and Uncle Carl, such as china, silver, crystal, etc. It had no sentimental value to her.

The following week, Uncle Ben and I visited the law firm in Oakland. I gave them copies of the pertinent files I took from Uncle Carl's desk. We were back in Stanislaus County the following week for the court case of the contested will. It was a shocker, a fraudulent and corrupt justice system.

The preacher lied as a witness, saying the $25,000 was a gift. He would not testify against Kathy. The Cadillac salesman allowed a $1,500 trade-in on a car with a low blue book of $8,500. He sold him a new Oldsmobile that was $4,000 over sticker price. Uncle Ben's attorney retained a retired district attorney to investigate criminal charges against Kathy for administering excessive medication. When he brought this up to the sheriff in Stanislaus County, they told him to "butt out." They would not investigate, and the DA had no jurisdiction. The witness at the bank who could verify that Kathy was taking items from the safety deposit suddenly disappeared. She no longer worked at the bank. Her mother had no idea where she was. The judge made the statement that the attorney who wrote the *new* will without reviewing it with Uncle Carl should be disbarred. The foreman of the jurors stated in court that they held hands and prayed that Kathy would win. Did Kathy move back to Wisconsin with her winnings? We heard from our sources that Kathy had moved to San Francisco and was caring for an elderly woman who was quite wealthy. Someday Kathy will make a mistake and be judged by her maker.

A lesson learned: a power of attorney is not worth the paper it's written on, and a joint will is of little value—at least in Stanislaus

County, California. To pour salt in Uncle Ben's wounds, his legal fees were a total of $17,000 before they went to court, which lasted two days. Earlier, he had sent the law firm a check for $15,000. At the end of the case, his balance was $49,000. In the beginning, the attorney gave Uncle Ben an estimate of "not to exceed $20,000." His final bill for legal fees was $64,000, and for what? It was a high price to pay to learn a lesson of a corrupt legal system that included an unscrupulous and unethical attorney who should have been disbarred, a judge who should have been removed from the bench, and a rigged jury. I'll throw in the sheriff's department who turned their back on a criminal investigation. Adding insult to injury, when I called the California Bar Association to complain about Uncle Ben's legal fees, they told me, "Tell your uncle to quit bitching and pay his damned bill."

TAKE ACTION

If you are involved with selecting a live-in caregiver for an elderly relative or friend, use extreme caution and exercise due diligence. One can never be too careful, as we learned in our situation with Uncle Carl. Uncle Ben thought he had all the bases covered. Are older people always the victim? Do they ever win?

CHAPTER 3

DIARY FROM 2005

The year was 2005. Twenty years had passed since our family had "diagnosed" my mother as being in the mild stage of Alzheimer's. Upon examination, three medical doctors had said Mom was simply getting senile and we should not be concerned.

My wife, Penny, was the office manager for an OB/GYN who had decided to retire. Both were 71. She had been with the doctor for 17 years. Insurance companies were her major source of stress. They "lost" most of their invoices, requiring second, third, and fourth copies of invoices. Then they would say she used the wrong coding, even though the coding was straight from their book. They dragged their feet on paying, 30 days stretching into 90 and more. This had been the norm for over 15 years, and now it was getting worse. Twenty-five percent of her time was wasted arguing with insurance companies. She trained the new hires—receptionists and medical assistants—as well as being responsible for the bookkeeping. Was the stress too much? I could not detect any early signs of Alzheimer's, but I saw her every day. Our daughters, who saw her at least once a week, said I was in denial. I clipped a magazine article about natural products and nutrition for Alzheimer's disease, thinking maybe they would help.

September 9, 2005. She's forgetful in the evenings after work. She drove to a shop not visited in many years with no problems. Without a computer she has no problems with daily bookkeeping. She has problems staying with the liturgy in church, keeps asking me where we are in the program.

October 2005. She apparently mailed out three payments that never arrived at their address. Is she forgetting to mail invoices to patients? Check and review with banks. I must watch her closely to see that she turns off appliances. At dinner, I prepared her plate with a baked potato, squash, and sauerkraut with sausage. She took a plate from the cupboard and cut up sausage from another piece for me, overlooking her original plate. I observed her trying to change channels with the remote. She was studying the remote as if she had no idea how to use it. There are times when I see her do something that indicates she's confused. However, within seconds she will do something indicating the contrary. Is it because she was *not concentrating* the first time? Being ADD, I'm guilty of that.

November 2005. During lunch, our waitress set her pepper shaker directly in front of my mom and she could not find it. She asked for the ground pepper mill, which she does not use ... not concentrating. She recognizes that she is forgetting, blames it on work. She has no problem with insurance company names, phone numbers, and patient files.

In early 2005, my wife was winding down the medical practice of her doctor, a gifted and compassionate OB/GYN. With the doctor being the same age as my wife, they continued past "retirement age" of 65 and now were both 72. But in late 2005 the malpractice insurance skyrocketed. The doctor had an enviable small practice where she continued doing the work she loved, bringing children into the world. She had patients from around the globe. Her expertise was therapy for infertility.

I crunched some numbers to see what the doctor was making as an income for her devotion to mankind. With more than 12 years of higher education, she was earning a little more than $18 an hour for her professional talents, while being on-call 24/7. An OB doctor was responsible for the mental and physical well-being of the child she delivered until 21 years of age. That's why their malpractice insurance is so high— more than a cardiologist. Someday a sharp attorney will convince a jury that an OB was indirectly responsible for a child's IQ.

It took about a year to close her practice. There were numerous forms to send out to all the patients in the past five years of files, notifying them of the closing of her office and practice. Dating back to 1953, the year my wife worked as a medical stenographer for a research doctor from New York, she had worked for five doctors. This would be her second "retirement planning" for a medical doctor. Being the office manager, she was a full-time bookkeeper, part-time receptionist, part-time medical assistant, and the instructor/trainer for the new receptionists and medical assistants. She was an impeccable bookkeeper, accurate to the penny. The doctor's CPA advised her, "When your office manager retires, you better fold your tent and retire."

In closing the practice, I helped her with the mailings and files. This is when I noticed she was sending out duplicate letters and invoices. Earlier, our daughters had noticed the changes in her behavior. A weekly visit makes it much easier to detect a change in behavior than my daily observation. When they brought it to my attention, I contacted my doctor, who was also her doctor. I wrote a note listing items that might be of concern. I requested our doctor to perform a preliminary examination that might lead to a more comprehensive exam by a doctor who specializes in dementia and geriatrics. Our doctor refused to give her an exam. When I tried to get a referral, I got the run-around. Finally, after much frustration and grief, I canceled our insurance with that provider and doctor.

My wife had a fantastic memory. From the day we married, she never had to write notes on the calendar to remind her of an anniversary or birthday for any member of the family. She could do the weekly shopping without a list. I hinted toward writing notes on the calendar, like the rest of us. She was a full-charge bookkeeper without the "crutch" of a computer. Try that sometime when you're paying business taxes...city, county, state, federal, plus all the other institutions with their hands out. Apparently, it become too much and her brain became overloaded.

The State Department of Motor Vehicles renewed her driver's license for another 8 years with no problems and no written exam. Her driving around Beaverton was excellent, no problems. However, I doubt if she could pass a written and/or a driving test. If she drives her memorized/routine route, she's okay. I tested her driving skills on an alternate route. She performed quite well, considering I put her through "one helluva test." When we got home in the driveway, I apologized to her for being rude in shouting out directions.

"I knew you were testing me," she said.

Debbie, our older daughter, has a BS in Nursing. She has her own business and worked out of her home as a medical examiner for insurance companies. Her husband, Robert, was employed by TriMet. Their three daughters, Ashley, 22, and the twins, Jaimie and Mandy, who were 19, lived nearby. Debbie, with her vast network in the medical sector, came up with a list of doctors who would take new, older patients who were on Medicare.

It took one year to locate and review new doctors.

Fortunately, we were in good health during the time we did not have supplemental insurance.

Penny was involved in a fender-bender in a bank parking lot. She told me about it upon returning home. When I asked her to explain what happened, she became confused. Assuming she was upset, I did not press the issue. Then she gave me a card with a woman's name and phone number—a witness. I called the witness to get her story. She confirmed that Penny had backed out of her parking spot and was stopped when the other car backed out and bumped her car. She said it was not Penny's fault. This was the same basic explanation Penny had given me. I filed an accident report and got an estimate from a repair shop. I asked the repair shop for their opinion on which car was at fault. They replied, "This is the most common fender-bender in a parking lot. We see them every day. From the location of the dent on the fender, your wife's car was stopped. The other driver backed into her car."

They are the experts in reconstructing the accident and I accepted their analysis. She still had problems explaining to me where she was parked, how she backed out, where the other vehicle was parked, etc. I was concerned about her losing her driver's license. I was also worried about her in an emergency at a busy intersection. Could she make the required split-second decisions? If she could not, she could be injured or injure someone else. Car damage is minor compared to bodily injury.

I got a good whiff of a potential problem with our insurance company. The other driver had the same insurance company. Over the years, I knew friends who'd had auto accidents, and if the other driver was insured by your company, you could be in for trouble. A red flag warning! If the accident was caused by the other driver, but they were a better client with greater potential for paying the insurance company more money because they had more cars, pickups, boats, homes, etc., the adjuster may deem it a "no fault accident." But it's different than if the other driver was at fault. The adjuster said, "Each driver is sharing fault." But it was not my wife's fault. Why should she share the fault? This statement from the insurance company would be a permanent note on her driving record. In her 57 years of driving, she had never had an accident. The witness confirmed that it was not my wife's fault. I phoned the witness to ask her what she told the insurance adjuster. Suddenly, the witness became hostile and refused to talk with me again. Had she changed her story? Not one to give up easily, I had means of checking the other driver's records—accidents, citations, etc. He'd had six moving violations in the past 18 months. When I called the adjuster to advise her of the other driver's driving record, she told me the case was closed and hung up on me. A pure case of politics trumping what actually occurred. It's called "business ethics."

Now that Penny had a new doctor, we asked her about having the Department of Motor Vehicles send my wife a form for a renewal test. She prescribed a better test, specifically designed for older people, that would not be sent in to DMV or their insurance company. If my wife failed the test, it was an indication she should give up driving, rather than wait for an accident. It's also a more compassionate method, preventing the family from becoming the "villain." The test was quite involved. I sat near her, but could not make comments that would help her score. I never saw her score, but I doubt if she achieved better than 50%. I seriously doubt if half of our society over 65 could achieve a score better than 70%. She reluctantly volunteered to give up the car and stop driving.

Next came the super-duper, full-blown, "Binford 9000" six-hour test performed by clinical psychologists in the area of neuropsychology. Various people on his staff administered the testing. I could not sit in to observe. She was totally exhausted from the testing ordeal, both mentally and physically. When we got home she went to bed without eating dinner. There were additional interviews where I could sit in. After reviews by other medical professionals and our doctor, she was diagnosed as being in the early stages of Alzheimer's disease. What we assumed a year prior was finally confirmed by a staff of medical professionals.

After the Food and Drug Administration (FDA) banned the importation of a highly successful high blood pressure herbal formulation from India, we had to resort to Western drugs. It took over two years of various prescribed medications to bring her high blood pressure down to normal. In the process, her kidneys and liver were stressed, almost damaged. With her thyroid being kept in check with medication, her doctor concentrated on Penny's borderline osteoporosis and high cholesterol. She was also taking a few typical herbal, mineral, and vitamin supplements. For memory, ginkgo biloba was added. After a few weeks, ginkgo was found to increase her blood pressure. I switched to gotu kola, which does not increase blood pressure. When Aricept, the most popular AD drug was prescribed, I hesitated. I had been researching on the internet for any herbal and mineral formulations that could help patients with AD.

An herb in Eastern Europe had been used as a memory enhancer for several decades—the snowdrop. The Europeans list medicinal herbs as drugs. The FDA also termed this European herb a drug. How interesting! An herb from Europe that has been used for decades to improve memory is now considered a "drug" by the FDA. After much hesitation, I had the Aricept prescription filled. The side effects were disastrous. Diarrhea! It was so bad, it literally oozed out of her while she was in bed sleeping. She woke up screaming and ran to the bathroom, leaving a messy trail behind her. She took a shower as I cleaned the bed, bedroom, and bathroom. She came back to bed and cried herself to sleep. The next morning she remembered her diarrhea incident. I did not say anything about the Aricept drug as being the culprit. She skipped Aricept a few days while I had her take a high-fiber supplement drink that solved the diarrhea problem for the moment.

I returned to the internet site that described an herbal product, the snowdrop (*Galanthus nivalis*). Its origin is the Caucasus Mountains (Russia, Turkey, Armenia, and Georgia) and Southern Europe.

It has also been found growing in gardens in Middle and Western Europe. The snowdrop develops from a small bulb that grows near the surface of the ground. Older people from the regions eat the bulbs to rejuvenate their brain and feel younger. Scientists from Bulgaria studied the snowdrop from the Caucasus Mountains and found the alkaloid galantamine. Western scientists developed a drug with artificial galantamine. Their rationale for a synthetic plant? Due to the large number of people with Alzheimer's, there were not enough snowdrop bulbs growing in the world. I wonder if they ever considered growing organic snowdrops as a farm crop in a domestic setting. With a patented (US patent 4,663,318) synthetic galantamine, the drug companies can sell their product at a higher price than an organic plant. They also control the market. However, the drug galantamine will have all the inherent side effects that are common with pharmaceutical chemical drugs. What are the typical side effects of the snowdrop growing in the wild? Maybe an upset stomach, if one overdoses.

On the drug information sheet, the side effects listed for galantamine are: "Nausea, vomiting, diarrhea, dizziness, loss of appetite, and weight loss may occur ... fainting, slow heartbeat, difficult urination, seizures, black/bloody stools, vomit that looks bloody or like coffee grounds, severe stomach/abdominal pains, irregular heartbeat ... an allergic reaction may include: rash, itching/swelling of the face/tongue/throat, severe dizziness, trouble breathing, aggressiveness. This is not a complete list of possible side effects." Also listed are numerous precautions based on your medical history.

December 2005. Penny's forgetting to mail out utility bill payments. She also has problems in church with Lutheran liturgy. If she loses her place, she has problems finding where we are in the program. If she loses her place in the hymnal, I show her and she continues until she loses it again. It's very small print. Her typical evening glass or two of wine becomes three or four. Is she forgetting how many she consumed? Although there are doctors who advocate the drinking of a couple cocktails, or wine or beers in the evening, Penny would consume in excess of moderation. Supplements (herbal, mineral, vitamins) lose their effectiveness when one consumes alcohol beyond moderation. The months of December and January were very hectic for Penny, closing the doctor's office. It seemed like all parties—insurance, suppliers, and city, county, federal, and state agencies—ceased to cooperate. The doctor only made the job more difficult. The doctor had the telephones shut off while they were still required in daily work. Their landlord pressured them to move out so it could lease the space, only adding to their stress. After they moved out, even though the office did not require remodeling, it remained vacant for six months.

February 2006. The next three months were spent reorganizing our home with an office. The doctor had given Penny her desk, copier, and fax machine from the office to continue the doctor's accounts receivable each month, mailing patient statements, etc.

May 2006. Her forgetfulness and negativity seemed to be getting worse each week. She feeds the dogs and forgets she fed them. She can maintain the patients' payment records and balance her personal checking account each month, but it takes longer. During our 50-plus years of marriage, I've never known her to lose her keys, purse, or anything of urgent need or value. I can't recall her bouncing a check or running out of gas in her car. How many of us can say that? Her secret? The fuel tank on her car never drops below one-quarter, her checking account balance seldom was below $1,000. Penny has revealed confusion in cooking and operating the dishwasher, clothes washer, and dryer. They are the new high-tech models with all the "bells and whistles" she insisted on having.

I have been taking gotu kola for many years to improve my

memory. I also perform math problems in my head. Seldom do I use a calculator to reconcile my bank account. In many cases my memory is as good as it was 30 years ago. We all have a problem with "brain overload"—it's common in our society. The older we get, the more data we store in our brain. I tend to "block entry" on some data to my brain. With our present technology there is no need to memorize vast knowledge. We can find it on the internet. Our brain should be used for thinking, rather than memorizing.

In our society, if a 50-year-old people have problems losing their keys, credit card, or remembering where they parked their car, it's blamed on stress and having "too much on their plate." However, when a 65-year-old person has these same problems, it's Alzheimer's. And yes, sometimes it is.

There may be a name for it—selective memory, maybe. She will ask me several times a day: "Did you make an appointment to have my car serviced?" She cannot remember that I told her several times that I made the appointment.

June 2006. Her weekly routine. We have walked two miles every day for the past 16 years. Monday, clean house, lunch at Honey Baked Ham; Tuesday, grocery shop at Costco and WinCo, lunch at Newport Bay; Wednesday, shopping at the mall, lunch at Newport Bay; Thursday, miscellaneous—wash clothes, pay bills; Friday, hair salon, lunch at Newport Bay. She drives her memorized route to the local shops and, as co-pilot, I observe her driving; it's as good as it was 30 years ago. When she parks in the mall, she always recalls where she parked. I have problems recalling where I parked.

Debbie called in a panic. "Mom, I can't find my car in the parking lot." A few weeks ago, she called me. "Dad, I can't find my cell phone." She was parked in downtown Portland. I asked her, "What are you calling on?" Her response? "Goodbye, Dad."

In our society, we do not focus on our present task. We day-dream and go through our routine, which I know includes talking on our cell phone while we're driving. There will be situations where the 50-year-old has Alzheimer's and the 65-year-old has too much on his or her plate, right? Multitasking is not good for our brain, according to the latest neurological research. There is a new phrase for performing a function, whether it's shopping, painting a room, driving to a new address, repairing a fence, etc. It's called "Computational Thinking." Most of us have done this all our life. We determine the steps required to complete a task, even something as simple as brushing one's teeth. However, in our modern society we have branded it with a name: more stuff to remember.

July 2006. She can count out her pills, drugs, and supplements as I observe, and put them in a plastic container that holds a week's supply. She stopped drinking wine for a few weeks. Her memory and attitude seemed to improve.

October 2006. I began reviewing new health and medical plans. Rumor has it that it takes a graduate from the law school at Yale, or a Philadelphia lawyer, to guide one through the health insurance and medical maze.

February 2007. Regence BlueCross BlueShield approved our enrollment, beginning February 1, 2007. Debbie and I began searching for doctors who would accept our insurance. We favored a doctor with an office in Northwest Portland who specialized in geriatrics with a background in Alzheimer's patients. Although her practice was closed to new patients, we convinced her to accept Penny. However, her earliest appointment date to see Penny was August 21, 2007, six months away. I found a new primary doctor and made an appointment for May 30, 2007. All of our medical records would be transferred to our new respective doctors.

June 2007. A visit to the ER at Legacy Good Samaritan hospital required an MRI. The results showed no damage, no signs of a stroke, etc. The new doctor prescribed drugs because of a borderline bone density issue that was revealed in the MRI. I added an herbal formulation for memory. She exchanged items at Macy's with the cleared check from the bank and sales receipt with no assistance from me. I drove 25 miles to visit with a grade school classmate I had not seen since 1945. Penny held a good, but limited conversation with the couple.

In July, we attended meetings of "Getting Started" at the Alzheimer's Association in NW Portland. For the next few weeks I contacted the main Alzheimer's Association, plus various state organizations. I asked for information on any group that had experience with herbal, mineral, and vitamin supplements (including formulations) that had shown promise with Alzheimer patients. Not one reply. I volunteered for a panel on AD, thinking I could add something to the group concerning our experience with memory and calming supplements. Again, not one reply. Periodically, I contact various AD groups in the US, concerning their experience with supplements. To date, I'm still waiting for a reply. The Big Three (American Medical Association, Food and Drug Administration, and Big Pharma) must have quite an influence on the AD associations.

These were her supplements prior to evaluation by her new doctor, for blood pressure, circulation, and memory: horse chestnut, motherwort, CoQ10, Vitamins C, B, D and E, lecithin, potassium, aspirin, calcium. Also, passionflower capsules and/or chrysanthemum tea for calming.

August 2007. At 2:45 a.m., in bed, she did not feel well. No headache, not dizzy, not sweating, but she could not explain how she felt. She seemed okay. Her blood pressure was 154/79, and her pulse was 66. Drank cold water, opened window for more cool air. Possibly gas; she began belching. Went back to sleep. 9:30 a.m., lying in bed. 11:00 a.m., blood pressure 121/61, pulse 63, relaxing, reading newspaper in lounge chair, reviewing old family photos. Walked for 15 minutes, cleaned and dusted until 12:45. Driving routine: once a week for shopping, approximately four miles on Highway 217—exact route every time, three times a week. She drives to Washington Square for shopping and lunch with friends, 1.5 miles. Friday, drives to hair salon. I ride with her at all times. She is a cautious and patient driver. A persistent cough required X-rays, which revealed no pneumonia, but the new doctor found chronic obstructive pulmonary disease (COPD). Additional medication required, including antibiotics.

September 2007. She follows along reading Lutheran liturgy and singing, and remembers where she parked the car. We attended a class reunion and caught up with the latest on our old classmates. She recognized a few, but they all knew her because of her red hair, tinted. It took her three hair stylists to find one who could duplicate her dark red hair to cover the gray.

October 2007. At Halloween, she enjoyed passing out candy to the youngsters and talking with them, like old times.

November 2007. She enjoyed the family gathering over Thanksgiving holiday. She likes to help clean up after meals; it keeps her busy. She's beginning to write more items on the calendar—appointments, birthdays, etc. We are watching her behavior closely. If we can control her aggressive behavior, the memory issue is of little concern. She has days of being "unruly" and having a chip on her shoulder. Medications help, but their side effects can present a problem. A periodic blood test will indicate if the drugs are stressing her system—kidneys, liver, etc. There are times when she has a blood test once a month in traversing that fine line.

December 2007. I suggested we not set up a Christmas tree this year. She agreed. We set up our village scene with lighted buildings. She wrote in a few Christmas cards for our relatives and close friends. I set up a small potted fir tree with a few ornaments to see if it met with her approval. She was polite and said it was okay. But when our granddaughter asked her how she liked it, she said, "It looks like crap." From our first Christmas tree in Oregon, she always had one of the best in the neighborhood.

February 2008. She has dreams that seem real to her. In the morning she questions me about people visiting or something that she recalls from her dream. At first, I would explain dreaming, which confused her. Then I changed the subject.

September 2008. I thought Penny fell asleep in the lounge chair. I tried to wake her to go to bed. She would not respond. Her pulse was very weak. I called 911 and then our daughter. Then my blood pressure spiked. The paramedics took both of us to ER. Penny finally came around. They drew her blood. While a nurse asked if she'd had anything to drink, Penny replied, "A glass of wine." The doctor making notes uttered to herself, "If she had blown a breathalyzer, it would have gone off the chart."

She had passed out from drinking too much wine. I had tried to watch her closely and limit her to no more than two glasses of wine. This time she fooled me and got more wine when I was not looking. She had been a heavy drinker since her early thirties. I considered her a borderline alcoholic, if there was such a term. At first it was hard liquor, then she favored wine. She never began drinking until evening, after work. In 1987, her daughters, a close friend, and a cousin called for an intervention to discuss her drinking. She never did admit she had a drinking problem. She could stop drinking for a couple months, then back to one glass of wine and eventually more.

Penny became very confused at Jaimie's wedding. Too many friends interacting with her, asking her what she wanted to do. "Go out to dinner ... spend time with a friend in Seattle ... visit a friend in Arizona ... visit her brother." I had to draw the line.

November 2009. She still writes checks and lists her DMV license number and telephone number on the checks from memory, although she does not drive. She marks each hymn listed by placing a donation envelope at the proper page in the

Lutheran hymnal. She continues to lose her place while singing when distracted. I show her the place to restart and she does okay until she gets distracted and loses her place again. This started about a year ago. Niko, our schnauzer, has diabetes. We began giving him insulin. Penny's very upset. When watching TV or reading in the lounge chair, Niko is cuddled with her. I placed one of Niko's antibiotic pills on the kitchen counter. Before I could turn back and get it Penny was right behind me, taking the pill from the counter and drinking water. This was the first time she had taken a pill from the counter. I always gave her pills in a shot glass. Never have I placed them on the counter. All of her pills are on the top shelf out of her reach, in a child- or AD person–proof container. I called poison control and was told it was harmless, but that it might give her an upset stomach.

December 2009. Numerous times she comes up to me with an embrace, telling me how much she loves me and thanking me for helping her. She addressed and wrote personal notes in twenty-five Christmas cards from a list I made, five at a time. I cross those names off and she writes another five. In church, she still recites the Apostle's Creed and the Lord's Prayer from memory. She finds her favorite TV programs in the *Oregonian* and checks off those she wants to watch, mainly comedy—*Frasier, Everybody Loves Raymond, The Golden Girls*. She cannot follow a TV drama or history. At Christmas, we displayed our village scene with the six lighted buildings, on a snow-covered table (cotton with a mirror) rather than decorating a small Christmas tree.

May 2010. When her doctor requested that she draw the hands on a clock showing ten minutes after nine, she could not do it. At home I spent 30 minutes with her trying to teach her how to tell time. She was patient, but I was quite shocked that she was now back to a three-year-old child. Her kidney function (BUN) and (creatinine) were over the high end of their range, indicating a drug-related problem, calling for a decrease in her high blood pressure medication. She had lab tests for bone density, a chest X-ray, and a mammogram. Doctor's office called to say they found her wrist watch. We thought she was imagining it, but she was right. She remembered losing it. Her doctor revised the dosage on her medication. I did the same with her herbal supplements. While shopping at Costco, she could not write the day or numerical amount on the check, only her phone number and DMV number.

October 2010. We switched doctors from downtown Portland to Beaverton, which was much closer. She is now seen by my doctor, who is in his sixties and is knowledgeable about Alzheimer's disease.

December 2010. After her bath, she became disoriented and felt dizzy. She dressed and changed to another outfit. While she was lying down on the bed I took her blood pressure. It was low. I called 911. Paramedics came and suggested we take her to ER for checkup after they ruled out heart problems. They suspected dehydration. A thorough checkup at ER confirmed dehydration and very low blood pressure. Her other vitals were okay. She was not drinking enough water. Her four glasses of iced tea per day had to be reduced to only two glasses. Tea is a diuretic. Indicators of a stroke did not exist. Her smile had a slight droop on one side. Her chin was warm, which indicated a possible tooth infection. A trip to the dentist and X-rays did not indicate any problems, other than a flare-up of a gum infection. That evening she had another incident of diarrhea. I told her she must stop drinking wine or she would continue to experience diarrhea. With no argument, she discontinued drinking wine. Her medication and supplements will have a better effect toward improving her health.

CHAPTER 4

DIARY FROM 2011

January 2011. She can't distinguish TV programs from commercials. She asks me to change channels, assuming I've got the TV on the wrong channel. January 13 was her worst day since being diagnosed. She was getting dressed for her hair appointment, but it was not Friday. It was our day for lunch at the Newport Bay restaurant. She would not sit down and relax with Niko. When she's not sitting with him, he jumps off the lounge chair and wanders through the house looking for her.

February 2011. I quit taking her grocery shopping. She gets too confused and can't keep up with me. She wants to check out items on the shelves of every aisle. I spend too much time trying to keep her near me. I can shop without her in half the time. She can't distinguish times of day or night. She may get up at 2:00 a.m. thinking it's time to take her bath and dress for lunch. She can still use the phone from a list in large type and read the newspaper. She frequently removes unwashed clothes from the washer and puts them in the dryer. She does this quickly, while I'm in the bathroom. She's like a child trying to get away with something she should not do. She plugged up the sink drain by pouring leftover oatmeal down the drain and washing away the evidence. That evening she put the leftover rice down the disposal. Days later, the drains stopped and I had to call the plumber. I've learned not to leave leftover food in the sink. Her nickname in the family is Miss Tidy Bowl. She was never one to leave dirty dishes in the sink. They must be rinsed and placed in the dishwasher. You must never leave your coffee cup with a couple swallows of warm coffee. She'll pour it down the sink drain and put the cup in the dishwasher.

March 2011. The least bit of interruption upsets her. A phone ringing or the door bell ringing upsets her for the remainder of the day. With a felt pen I write a list of the most important things for her to review each day and tape it on a cupboard door. Notes on the calendar only confuse her. She does not know the week or day or if it's daytime or nighttime. If I tell her, she cannot remember.

April 2011. Niko died on the 9th at 11:30 p.m. with his head on her pillow in bed. She was asleep with her hand on his front shoulder. Having diabetes, kidney and bladder infections, as well as being blind placed him close to the end of his life. Years before, I asked her if she wanted Niko to be put to sleep by our vet or to let him die at home, unless in pain. She preferred him to be home. I knew the day had arrived. His organs were shutting down. When he was happy (insulin shot daily, blind, with a bladder infection—what's to be happy about?) he would wag his tail when I talked to him and stroked under his chin. He stopped wagging his tail. When they went to bed, I placed his head on her pillow and checked on him every 30 minutes. By 9:00 p.m., they were asleep. His heart beat was weakening, his breathing was normal. Checking every half hour indicated he was slowly dying, with no pain. By 10:30, his heartbeat was very weak, his breathing was shallow, and his nervous system was going. Finally, there was no more life in Niko. Penny was sleeping. Gently, I took him away. She woke up from the movement and asked me where I was taking him. When I told her he was gone, she screamed and began crying. I placed him on a small rug in the spare bedroom. Neither of us slept the remainder of the night. She kept repeating, "He was my baby boy." Niko was twelve, a small, miniature schnauzer, black with a gray beard and gray feet. He only weighed 14 pounds. When he was eight weeks old we took him to the beach. He was so tiny, the runt of the litter. A man offered us $1,000 for him, finally raising his offer to $4,000. We would never sell him. We raised him from a runt with Penny feeding him with a bottle. He was not strong, but he protected Penny with his life, by being very aggressive around big dogs. He walked with us on our two-mile walks for years, until I had to carry him.

On the 14th, she went to bed at 7:00 p.m. to watch TV with Max, our younger miniature schnauzer, who tipped the scales at 24 pounds. A couple hours later, Max trotted out to the living room, excited. Then Penny walked out almost in tears.

"Niko fell off the bed and I can't find him." I took her back to bed and told her I would find him. Within 30 minutes, I went to bed and we watched TV for an hour. She never mentioned Niko again. She may have had a bad dream about Niko. By not explaining to her that Niko had died, I avoided her reliving his death, which would only bring back more pain and suffering.

May 2011. Our doctor increased Penny's anxiety drug (citalopram) to two pills a day—9:00 a.m. and 2:00 p.m. She's doing much better. I tend to give/take less prescription medication, due to their side effects. She's okay with one pill, but family stress increases her anxiety level. Every Saturday she dusts the furniture. She may dust the same table four times. She only signs one check after I write it—to Dennis, her hair stylist. My main problem as a caregiver is with her meals—no sandwiches, soups, or salads (at home). For lunch she will only order the pear/pecan/chicken salad at Newport Bay restaurant. She has been eating there for the past 20 years. Most of the servers know she has AD, but they have always treated her like a queen. When she was working for the OB/GYN, their crew lunched at NB four days a week. For dinner she enjoyed their grilled salmon or halibut.

There are times when we are out shopping that she may display her condition. As her husband and caregiver, I feel like placing a sign on her that reads: "Bear with me, I have AD."

I tend to be overprotective. I always have been. When I mentioned to a stranger that Penny was in the early stage of Alzheimer's, they replied, "I would never have known unless you told me."

She will not eat a frozen (she calls them boxed) meal of fish or chicken. Italian and Mexican food are out, unless you put it on her plate and tell her it's something else. Our daughters keep telling me to do what's best for me, so I don't burn out. It's difficult to do when the patient is your wife. I still ask her, "What would you like for lunch (or dinner)." She doesn't know. She can't answer. I'm slowly learning not to ask. She had a mild outburst in church. We always arrive early to get "our place" in the back of the church. Another couple have "their place" in front of us and are short so we have no problems seeing over them. This morning, they did not attend and a visiting couple took their place, but they were taller. She voiced her disapproval by being ornery. To calm her, I change the subject to distract her. Most of the time it achieves its purpose.

If only the medical doctors would have examined her a year earlier, as I suggested, she may not have progressed so far into another phase of AD.

If you suspect that a loved one in your family may be in the early stages of Alzheimer's, take action. Do not hesitate.

June 7 will be our 59th wedding anniversary. Here's how we celebrated:

June 6. After her breakfast of Swiss Miss cocoa with my secret recipe bran muffin with walnuts, plus cereal and fresh strawberries floating in half & half, it's pill time. I turned on her favorite TV programs. In the mornings, it's either *The Golden Girls* or *Frasier.* This morning it was *Frasier.* During my 20- to 40-minute break, I'll add a few lines to my next book project, or edit *Laughter and Tears.* At 10:00 a.m. I switch the TV to *Everybody Loves Raymond* DVDs. This will allow me up to an hour to beautify our yard. This year will be a chore ... edging the front yard shrub beds and applying an additional layer of bark dust. Too bad parents can't teach their youngsters how to care for lawns and yards. I would hire out the work, but they don't do the work to my satisfaction, even though I tell them and show them. I guess they're in too much of a hurry to get home and play video games on their computer. I had a quick lunch and turned on a TV program for Penny while I did a bit of yard work. After an hour, I came back in the house to make sure she had something to keep her busy, like emptying the clothes dryer and putting our clothes in their drawers. She can also empty the dishwasher and put the items in their proper place, but not always. It gave me time to grocery shop at a local supermarket. When I returned I found her in the kitchen "drying" her freshly polished fingernails over the red-hot burner on our ceramic stove top. The burner was on high! I was upset with her, but she denied she had turned on the burners. AD patients don't know what they have done. She walked out to the living room to watch a program on TV. While I was putting the groceries away, I was mad at myself. I tell myself that from now on if I'm gone for a few minutes I must turn off the range at the power panel. Unless I'm running a load of clothes through the wash, I will unplug the power cord. She may wash one item when I'm not nearby. It's as if they are a child wanting to do something they know they should not. If it's random, why don't AD patients do something that you want? And why do AD patients display anger rather than a less aggressive emotion? I'm sure when I read more about the human brain, I'll find the answer.

June 7, 2011. After her breakfast we talked about lunch and dinner for the week. We discussed dinner tonight at our favorite restaurant. Our daughters called to wish us a happy anniversary. Penny can make our queen size bed. This morning I helped her. She feeds Max and rewards him with a treat. Her typical morning includes throwing the ball for Max to retrieve. Many days, she does this two or three times. It's good exercise for them. On nice days, I throw the ball for him in the back yard until one of us becomes exhausted. Debbie and Robert took us to lunch. Our granddaughter Ashley joined us for a delightful late lunch that would put our dinner on hold until Friday. Back home, Penny arranged the outfit she would wear for lunch the next day. It was back to the routine of playing ball with Max and watching TV. I continued working in the yard, checking on her every 15 minutes. I picked a bouquet of irises from our garden and Ashley brought us a bouquet of peonies. Penny never mentioned our anniversary again. We enjoyed a light supper and I turned on the TV to the *Glenn Miller Story*. When it came to the scene where his orchestra played "In the Mood," I said, "There's our song." Penny got up from her lounge chair and danced around the room for Max and me. She remembered.

Over the past 60-plus years I have recalled her energy and vibrancy in high school. She was in every sports activity, on the rally squad, and a majorette. In her business courses she received high honor awards in bookkeeping, shorthand, and typing. She had a column in the high school paper—"In the Husky Den with Pen." Upon graduation she received a scholarship in journalism to the University of Oregon, which she never pursued.

We were married a year later. Penny loved to dance. She could have been a professional ballroom dancer. I took dancing lessons just trying to keep up with her. Her first work experience after high school was in sales at a department store, then a car hop at the Red Head Drive In. The owner's two daughters were red heads. Her first plunge into the business world was with a bank. After a few months, Penny was lured away with a higher salary to become the receptionist and full charge bookkeeper for a Chevrolet dealership. Under the model of the strict General Motors Acceptance Corporation accounting system, she gained valuable lifetime experience. While with me in the military in Georgia she was the medical stenographer for a research doctor from New York who had a laboratory in Augusta. During her working career she was in women's high fashion sales for a department store. She returned to her passion of working for doctors (five) and caring for their patients. She learned to give injections, take blood pressure, and perform other patient functions to assist the doctors. She taught me how to give injections to our daughter for her allergies.

We enjoyed an evening of cocktails and dancing in clubs around Portland and on the Oregon coast. With me being challenged with ADD, various dancing steps became quite an effort. With swing being our favorite dance, it was difficult for me to develop a routine that I could duplicate. I developed an unorthodox swing style and Penny followed perfectly, making me appear as if I knew what I was doing. In a couple clubs in Portland, other dancers thought we were professionals. A couple clubs in our hometown, one on the Oregon coast and two in Portland, would play our "theme song" when we arrived for an evening of dancing. "Pennies from Heaven" was our cue to dance. If they really wanted the crowd to shuffle onto the dance floor they played "In the Mood." It was our cue to break the ice and be cool.

Our greatest dancing performance was in the main ballroom at the Hilton Hawaiian Village in Honolulu. It was during our 25th wedding anniversary trip. Our daughters pooled their resources and gave us a wing-ding of a send-off party in Portland, plus over a week on Kauai, Maui, and Oahu. While on Oahu, we began an evening in a small bar at the Hilton, dancing to their jazz combo until they closed. The barmaids encouraged us to continue our dancing in their main ballroom. Dancing to a 16-piece orchestra was awesome. As the evening progressed we danced to all of our favorite steps—the cha-cha, rumba, samba, and swing. It seemed like the orchestra leader was challenging us with each number, a different dance step. When the orchestra began Glenn Miller's "In the Mood," it struck a chord within us. It was our cue to perform, to do our best in front of a ballroom crowd of at least 300 people dressed to the nines in gowns and dinner jackets. Halfway through the number we noticed the other dancers were not dancing, allowing us more room—the entire ballroom floor. Penny was never lovelier with her long, dark red hair, a yellow "aloha" blouse and white shorts. I was dancing with my Queen. When the music stopped, "our audience" applauded and the orchestra leader bowed. We were quite embarrassed. We were not dressed in formal or even semi-formal attire. We ran from the ballroom, feeling as if we were captured in a "Cinderella" moment. The pedi-cabs were not operating. Penny was exhausted, and her feet were sore. I carried her piggyback for a few blocks back to our hotel. We paid for our dancing the following morning with sore feet. Thanks to my photographic memory, I can still picture her that evening.

It has taken Penny over five years to progress into the moderate stage of AD. With my research into alternative medicine and the drugs that medical science has developed, I'm gambling and praying that she will remain in the moderate stage and not progress into the advanced stage of AD. It would take a miracle in medical science to reverse the conditions of AD, but I'm not ruling it out.

July 2011. Currently, for AD only, she takes the following products: Medication—galantamine, 24 mg; Supplements—herbal, mineral, and multivitamin formulations. Many are proprietary. Our health insurance will not pay a dime toward our supplements, only the drugs. Our cost for her brain-enhancing supplements is less than $100 per month. Our cost, in addition to our insurance premiums, for her medications is less than $100 per month.

She was in good spirits all week. Being one who loved to shop for bargains, she scanned all the advertisements from mailers and the newspaper. Much like a child cutting out paper dolls, she has clippings of jewelry, bathroom rugs, shoes, gifts, flowers, etc., that she squirrels away in her purse. Recently, I gave away 60 years' accumulation of jewelry to our granddaughters and daughters. She had at least a dozen pairs of sunglasses. From a mailer, she found a pair of shoes she wanted—to add to her more than ten pairs in her closet. I gave twenty pairs to Goodwill. I discarded most of the mailers and newspapers into recycling, hoping she would forget. We enjoyed lunch on Wednesday and Friday with no disappointments or noisy patrons with unruly Katzenjammer Kids sitting nearby. Sunday evening we celebrated our wedding anniversary with a grilled seafood dinner. This was the first time in years that she ate their Parmesan mashed red potatoes with herbs. She never noticed. Instead of her usual glass of wine, she had iced tea. I did not order a drink. Over the years my favorite drink had switched from scotch to Bailey's Irish Cream. Just in the past week, Penny has favored country-western music over her past favorites—big bands, classical, and jazz—which she picked up from me. Our collection included the greats: Dave Brubeck, Paul Desmond, Ella Fitzgerald, Miles Davis, Gerry Mulligan, Oscar Peterson, and George Shearing. Finally, she watched old classic movies on TV like *The Snows of Kilimanjaro, Love Is a Many Splendored Thing,* and *An Affair to Remember.* I slipped in a *Dirty Harry* (Clint Eastwood) DVD, but she considered it too violent. Monday was a sad day for me. I spent 30 minutes trying to teach her how to read time on a clock. When the "big hand" is on a number she thinks it's that time. I was explaining that the "little hand" must be on the number. After the 30 minutes, she said, "I don't understand." Many times in the past, if I explained something to her or corrected her (which I stopped doing), she would get upset and go to our bedroom saying, "I know I'm dumb and stupid."

It's difficult for me to accept. After all these years of being an intelligent woman, she has regressed to the point of not being able to tell time. I have a difficult and challenging task before me.

August 2011. We took a day trip to Seattle with Debbie and Robert to visit our great-grandsons and Penny's brother. Jack will be two in October. Henry is three weeks old. We toured West Seattle in Jaimie's SUV. With the two young boys it was not a good day to tour the shops in the Pike Place area. We lunched at a seafood restaurant on the waterfront. Although Penny missed lunching at Newport Bay in Portland, she "survived" with a Cajun chicken salad and iced tea.

Typical young boy that he was, Jack's interest on the carousel took a "flirting" detour to a little blond girl with long curls. The warm Puget Sound afternoon was fading. It was nearly time to pick up Jaimie's husband at Nordstrom. Back at their home in West Seattle, we spent more time with the boys before visiting Penny's brother Ed in Renton.

After being a snowbird in Yuma, Arizona, for years, he was not able to return to the desert this year. Within the past few years, Ed had suffered serious cardiovascular problems. He'd had bypass surgery, plus numerous stents. Penny was quite upset when she saw him the previous fall when he'd returned from Yuma. The six-foot-three, 220-pound ex–high school star quarterback, power forward and outfielder was down to a mere 160 pounds. With his family's support, he consented to check into an assisted living facility. His son was visiting when we arrived. We toured the facility while they had dinner. Back in his room, with my coaching, Penny reminisced with Ed about their more pleasant youthful days in northern Minnesota. You could sense the bitterness in Ed, who did not favor living in what he called "an assisted living compound." At 75, he still had his sharp, witty mind. He was a fun, party guy earlier in his life. It had been a long day. Penny did very well, considering. Since that day, she has mentioned her brother many times.

"I'm glad I got to visit with Eddie. He does not look well. I don't think he'll make it much longer."

Rather than agree with her, I brought up their memories. We have his graduation pictures from high school and college among others in our living room. Now and then, as she passes either picture she says, "He was sure a handsome young man."

"Still is, but like the rest of us, he has a few more wrinkles," I reply, and she smiles.

I keep reminding her that Ed has a nice apartment, his son and daughter live nearby, and he is receiving very good care and healthy meals. Ed's idea of a healthy meal was a Whopper, French fries, and a Coke. Oh, and occasionally, a couple shots of Wild Turkey. When we were visiting, it was wine tasting and socializing night at the "compound." Until he can organize a group in his new "compound," Ed will miss his old geezer "hold 'em" poker gang in Yuma.

Our brain is such a complex mass of tissue and stuff that I may never understand it. Penny will ask the same question numerous times, but not remember that I gave her an answer. She will attempt to phone her hair stylist numerous times to make an appointment for a perm, but not remember that I left a message for him to call. Why is it they can remember one situation, but not another? Apparently, her brain does not transfer their incoming calls to storage for later retrieval. The scientists claim it's the plaque that puts up a roadblock for the transmitters.

We visited my cousin's open house honoring their 60th wedding anniversary. Penny did quite well, considering. When she started telling the same story repeatedly, I tried to alter the situation by prompting her to bring in another subject. Her favorite story was leaving Minneapolis and moving to Oregon. I added that she left a city of 300,000 to settle in a logging town of 1,500. She does okay when I prompt her to talk about her ice skating and her interest in fashion design in grade school, attending plays, concerts, operas, and so on. When she gets to the point of searching for a word, I can prompt her to reduce potential frustration. She does not get upset with me. We're like a comedy team. At the open house we enjoyed light finger food, cake, and punch.

On our return trip to Beaverton, we stopped in Seaside for a light supper. Penny had become quite fussy about her food— no Italian or Mexican, no soups or sandwiches. Chinese was her favorite, but now it's low on her acceptable list. She will not eat a salad that I prepare at home. As we entered a Mexican restaurant, she refused to go inside until we told her she could order a salad. She would only eat the chicken from her taco salad. However, she did eat part of my chili rellenos. A few years earlier, her favorite meals that I prepared were beef or chicken stir fry with veggies; a hearty beef stew; stuffed peppers; and grilled halibut and salmon. Chicken teriyaki with wild and brown rice or red potatoes became one of her favorites. For snacks she enjoyed apples, oranges, peaches (in season), and fruit yogurt.

"I'm tired of wearing my pajamas and watching TV. Let's go for a drive," I say. I needed metal buttons for my logger's suspenders that attach to my work jeans. I'll take her with me. She dressed and we were on our way. As we entered the store, I asked a sales lady for directions. What she told me was wrong. As we walked down various isles, Penny was grabbing items from racks and shelves. "I need this, I want this." She was picking up buttons, hair pins, framed pictures, and stuffed animals, which I had to put back. As we were in line for check-out, she grabbed a calendar. When I told her we had enough at home, she threw it toward the rack. By now, she was akin to a spoiled child, giving me the "stink eye." When we passed the candy section, she grabbed a candy bar. When I told her to put it back, she threw it to the floor. I'm now the mean parent and she will not stand near me. Walking out to our car, she walked in the middle of the traffic lane, until I reached for her arm to guide her to our car. Back in the car, she insists that we go to Newport Bay for lunch. In her mind, she wanted to go for a drive, knowing she could possibly talk me into taking her to lunch—a real con artist. I drove home.

Incoming mail as well as outgoing mail adds to her confusion. Our mail delivery route is a training route, so we receive our mail as early as 9:30 a.m. and as late as 5:30 p.m. I try to be in the house when the mail is delivered. Times when I'm not, the mail either disappears or I find it in the closet, in the cupboard with dishes, or wherever. When I receive the mail, I go through it looking for letters from friends, bills, and important stuff. All junk mail is placed in a stack for Penny and recycling. She goes through the junk mail and fills out coupons to all the solicitations for million-dollar deals, reverse mortgage con artists. She fills in her name and nothing else.

Outgoing mail can be quite different. If I mail a bill payment from the house, I put it out when I see the mail delivery truck down the street. One day, she took our outgoing mail and brought it back in the house, including three pieces that contained checks. She opened the envelopes, removed the checks and brought them to me with such a lovely smile to show me the checks we had received. Bless her heart. I smiled and thanked her. Large checks that I mail (most of our bills are paid online) are taken to the PostalAnnex next to her hair salon every Friday.

CHAPTER 5

DIARY FROM 2012

We spent a quiet evening at home New Year's Eve watching world events unfold on TV. Penny's brother had been in a Yuma hospital for a week. Tubes were required to drain fluid from his lungs. Penny's daughter Michele flew to Yuma to visit Ed. It was too much stress for us to go, but Penny talked with Ed on the phone. His son and daughter flew to Yuma. His many tubes were removed and a pump installed. For the next two days Penny became agitated at night. She wanted a bath, followed by dressing at 10:00 pm. Our favorite restaurant closed for remodeling. Penny had her first chicken sandwich from Arby's in more than 10 years, and she enjoyed it. A few days later, we tried Arby's French Dip sandwich. I did not mention it was a sandwich. I told her it was our French Dip lunch.

Mid-January 2012. We had a skiff of snow which turned into a blizzard for 15 minutes. Ed was failing. His blood pressure was 80/40, and his pulse was 42. His family tried to fly back to Yuma. With a power failure and light snow in the Northwest there were no flights to Yuma. By now, Ed was in a coma and not eating. A fourth day of snow was followed by rain. Winds were 50 to 70 mph on coast, with hurricane gusts to 110 mph. We had our first lunch, by personal invitation, at the newly remodeled restaurant. They had eliminated Penny's favorite items—pecan, pear, blue cheese salad, and Marionberry cobbler. She did not approve of their substitute, which was peach cobbler.

January 23. Penny went to bed in a good mood at 6:30 p.m. to watch TV. I checked on her and Max every half hour. By 7:30 she was asleep, and it was my time to rest and collect my thoughts of the day and prepare for tomorrow. I dozed off about 10:00. Max trotted out from the bedroom and the hall light came on. Penny was out of bed, fully dressed! It took an hour of diplomacy to convince her it was not time for lunch.

January 24. Ed died in his sleep. His ladyfriend in Yuma had a memorial at their resort park for their friends and his poker gang. Family will have their memorial in Renton in March. Penny knew her brother was failing. She mentioned he did not look well the last time they visited.

March 2012. Light snow during first week of the month. We took a road trip to Renton with Michele for Ed's memorial. I talked to the group about my salmon fishing and deer hunting trips with Ed, great times, great memories. Penny was in a good mood. She began a new regimen of herbal formulations for improving memory along with natural antibiotics. For relaxing and calming, she took the herb passionflower, as necessary.

April 2012. Penny had some dental work and was relaxed. The passionflower is working very well. She has no understanding of basic instructions—how to dress, how to brush her teeth, how to wash her hands. When I put liquid soap in her hand she does not know what to do with it. She does not know articles of clothing—sweaters, slacks, socks, etc.—I must show her. She can still operate the remote for TV channels with two digits and can sign her name.

I will monitor the 16 mg dosage of galantamine for 30 to 60 days. (Snowdrop, the natural galantamine found in European forests has no side effects.) Her first doctor (an Alzheimer's expert) had her on the 24 mg dosage—the highest—in two weeks. Other doctors suggest 8 mg for four weeks, 16 mg for four weeks, then 12 mg twice daily, sometimes 24 mg in a single dose.

May 2012. Bad day for Penny. She had a bowel movement accident in the bathroom, requiring a new toilet seat and cover. She did not realize what she had done. She has half a dozen outfits of various colors, but she'll only wear brown. Chocolate slacks, bra, panties, camisole, with a camel sweater. When it came time to wash, she would not wear any other color—not even her pajamas and robe—until her brown ones were washed and dried. Debbie convinced her to wear her black slacks and chocolate sweater. Now she has three sets of her brown outfit. She had a bad day. She rushed home from Debbie's (they live next door), pushing Debbie as she hurried out the front door, throwing her gloves at me. Very confused. She'll only watch TV if I join her. For the first time, she could not sign her name to a check. She asks me constantly: "Do we go to Newport Bay today?"

May 6. A better day. Penny watched TV and did not ask for a latte. She kept telling me she was sorry. On May 7, she got out of bed at 5:15 a.m.—too early—but was in good spirits.

May 8. Very stubborn this morning. Sat on the bed, half dressed, until her brown slacks were washed and dried. After that, she was in good spirits. Cutting her visits short at Debbie's after her latte, wanting to get home to be with Max.

May 9. Doctor refused to renew prescription for citalopram. He told the pharmacy her need was discontinued in November. Wrong. At her last appointment in November, we asked for an increase in citalopram to reduce her irritability. At that time he added trazodone for anxiety. The pharmacy filled the new prescription for trazodone and refilled the citalopram. We will seek a new doctor due to the current one having memory problems himself. Until we get a refill of citalopram, I will try an additional trazodone. The passionflower herb has been working well; it calms her, and she sleeps better. On sunny days, I work outside trimming and nurturing my baby trees, and weeding. Penny sits in a rocking chair in the garage with doors open to watch me. She reads and looks at pictures in books and magazines.

Week of May 20. Penny had moments of peace followed by being irritable. She does not like to change into pajamas and go to bed at night. She says she'll stay up until Wednesday when we go to lunch. It may take an hour of convincing to get her to go to bed; then she's mad. Another very bad day. I left her watching TV with Max to allow me time to tidy up the bathroom off our bedroom. As I passed the utility room on my way to the living room, I sensed a foul odor. She had a bowel movement on the floor of the utility room and her clothes. She was attempting to wipe up the mess with a soiled bath towel. She did not realize she had made the mess. This was the second time she did not use the bathroom. I did not scold her. She had another bath and told me she loved me. These are the tough days one must forget. She can tell me when she feels the urge to pee, but not a bowel movement.

I finally discovered a solution. When she sits to pee, I ask her to cough. It works every time; she has a bowel movement. It may not work with other AD people, but it's worth a try. Much depends on water intake, type of food, and time of day.

June 2012. Our granddaughters (Ashley, Jaimie, and Mandy) took Penny shopping for a new dress for our 60th wedding anniversary celebration. Ashley was the only one who could convince Penny to wear her new ivory dress for our special occasion. We were the center of attraction when our entourage entered the Skamania Lodge for brunch. The men were in dark suits sporting sunglasses on a bright morning in Washington. Were they the Columbia River Mafia? The day went well for Penny. She never had an incident. We closed out our anniversary brunch with the photographer taking numerous family pictures of the event.

We had our first appointment with our new doctor, a young woman, maybe in her late twenties or early thirties. She renewed Penny's citalopram prescription and drew blood.

Week of June 17. Michele picked us up for a Father's Day dinner at her home. Penny enjoyed the outing. However, she was constipated for five days. I assume it must be her drugs' side effects. I gave her a special herbal tea, but it worked too well. The next day she had another accident in the utility room. A real mess—rugs, towels, floor, clothes—another bath. My new procedure is not 100% effective.

Week of June 24. My doctor appointment (I also switched to Penny's new doctor) for annual checkup. In the doctor's office Penny became quite irritated and sassy. She's ready for bed from 8:30 on. The pills seem to be working. New doctor says the trazodone drug is more of a sleeping pill. She's okay dressing for bed now, no complaints. Medication and herbs seem to be balanced and working well. She did become a little agitated when she did not get color in her hair. Her color appointment is next week.

July 2012. Reviewing adult foster home facilities for Penny. Some nights I may get two hours of sleep. It's starting to have an effect on me. My doctor says the caregivers must become the care supervisor or they will burn out. My mother and Penny's mother were in adult foster homes rather than a nursing home. From the lists we had, it was vital that we check out the facilities we favored for any violations from city, county, state, or federal agencies.

CHAPTER 6

PREPARE FOR THE ROAD AHEAD

One week in August 2012—Highly stressful for everyone: We investigated an adult foster home in Wilsonville. Relatives of the owners/managers had an adult foster home nearby. State records checked out. We reviewed the home and saw that the operation did not have any residents with Alzheimer's. Penny would be their first. We moved her in on a Monday. She was quite upset. We brought her back home Wednesday. The owners lied to us. Their home was not a level-3 facility. They did not provide 24/7 nursing care. There was no manager awake at night to ensure a resident did not get up and wander. We found out the other two residents were tied in bed and given a sleeping pill. Thursday we reviewed a large memory home care facility in Oregon City. The marketing director assured us they were a level-3 facility with a 24/7 nursing staff. She was in her "new home" by Friday afternoon. We were advised not to visit or call her for two weeks.

Week of August 26. Penny is doing very well, not asking to go home, sleeping very well. After a week, Michele talked with her on the phone. She asked Michele to take her home, said people (residents) were weird, crazy. Michele called the next evening. She did not recall their phone conversation of the day before. Michele visited Friday afternoon. Penny's ankles were swelling. Too much walking? My first visit was on the first day of September. She was very happy to see me and was laughing and smiling. She did not ask to go home. Thank you, Lord.

Week of September 2. Penny had an excellent day on Sunday and was happy and smiling. She followed an aide around, assisting in light chores.

My Monday visit revealed ankle and leg swelling. Losing items—two pair of slacks, blouses, teddy bear, moisturizing cream, etc. Mouthwash had not been opened. She was happy to see us, and laughed. We sat outside, watched a movie, and snacked on pears. Debbie will call doctor about the swelling.

There was no nurse on duty. They lied to us.

Tuesday. Doctor asked us to bring Penny in at 12:30 p.m. The swelling was increasing. The doctor did tests, including an electrocardiogram, took a chest X-ray, drew blood, and gave us a prescription for Lasix to help deal with the edema, which she was experiencing for the first time in her life.

Thursday. Doctor appointment at 12:30 p.m. She had gained weight due to a mix-up with diuretic pills. I took a photo of feces on the shower floor; it was the third day without cleaning. Received the diuretic pills at our home address. Weird pharmacy.

Friday. I visited and delivered Lasix pills to the medical aide. The swelling was down. Placed her in a recliner with her feet elevated. Found out one of their "nurses" was terminated.

Saturday. I visited with our granddaughter, Mandy. Swelling was down. An ulcer was forming over her left ankle bone. She has lost four pounds.

Monday. Debbie and I took Penny to doctor's appointment. A new doctor suggested moving her to a better home. According to the State of Oregon, this was one of the best. No TED (compression) hose. They promised delivery in one day, and it's been three. I drove her to the pharmacy, bought the TED hose which they put on her right leg, not the leg with the wound...after I had told them which was the correct leg. The pharmacy had no order from the home. The home lied! Back at the home, an aide or nurse would put the compression hose on the correct leg.

September 17. No one at the home could draw blood per our doctor's request. They had to admit they did not have a nurse (RN) on staff. We would have to wait until the nurse visited next week. I took Penny to a Quest lab where they drew her blood.

September 24. Pharmacy nurse came by to draw blood, a week late.

October 8. HealthCare (a national firm) called me concerning "home care" for wound dressing. The MemHome's Resident Care Coordinator was back on duty from vacation. They did not want the responsibility for wound care, so they retained HealthCare. However, HC would not comply with our doctor's orders. The RC Coordinator suggested that I permit them to treat Penny, regardless of the fact that their wound care was unacceptable to our doctor. I told them they were foolish to make such a request.

October 9. We took Penny to doctor's appointment. She weighed 135.8 pounds, the heaviest she'd been in her life. Doctor again advised moving her. We began our search for a smaller facility, an adult foster home with a 24-hour Registered Nurse on staff.

October 11. Michele and I visited. HC visited to dress wound. We looked for other TED hose to put on left leg. No one could find it.

October 12. I visited and found the wound dressing was off and no TED hose. We were getting furious with their incompetency—from the head honchos down to the skivvy honchos (sub-bosses) and many of their aides, all idiots. Is it intentional? I found one who took personal care and provided proper attention to Penny.

October 13. I visited and found an "aide" dressed in black, tending to the wound. She dressed it in gauze and tape which stuck to the open wound. *Damn idiots.* We must watch them like a hawk, looking over their shoulder every minute. Both the Mem-Home and HC denied any of their people changed the wound dressing. Weird.

October 14. I visited and found no wound dressing, only a sheer stocking that had stuck to the wound scab. It seemed as if no one cared that they were not following our doctor's orders. Were they waiting for a lawsuit?

October 16. We visited and found wound covered with gauze and tape. We took photos and removed it. It had a bad odor. We put on dressing from HC then put on TED hose over wound. No problem.

October 17. I arrived at 2:15 p.m. There was no cover over wound and no TED hose, but she was in good spirits. She was dozing off in a swing-rocker in the activity room with many residents and aides. I left at 3:45. A medical aide called when I got home to say Penny had fallen out of the rocker. This is getting to be like the old "Keystone Kops" cartoons. They checked and found no pain.

October 18. A medical aide said Penny was sleeping on a makeshift bed on the floor when they went in to wake her. She had been there all night. She woke up active and in good spirits. HC dressed the wound—no TED hose—and wrapped ankle.

October 19. When I arrived at 10:00 a.m., she was asleep in her room alone. No wrap, wound dressing, or TED hose. Would this "high and mighty" MemHome facility treat an animal with such incompetency?

October 20. Relatives visited with Debbie—no wrap, wound dressing, or TED hose.

October 21. Michele found her asleep in the activity room in the lounge chair. I arrived at 4:00 p.m. and left at 6:30. Swelling of left ankle and leg was near normal. Her weight was 131. Medical aide said she would not take her meds since morning. At suppertime she took a few. Complained about hurting when trying to stand and walk. She could not move her feet until we "pulled" her shoulders. Left her in wheelchair and told caregivers. Ankle and wound were wrapped and dressed, no TED hose. Moved her legs to test for pain—none.

October 22. Debbie and I arrived at 2:00 p.m. Penny could not stand or walk without pain. We took her to the Willamette Falls Hospital emergency room. Her blood pressure was 83/37. They put her on IV fluids for five hours. The ER doctor and two supervisor RNs said if we had not brought her in she would not have made it through the night. Although her blood pressure was low, the med aides had not called her doctor for a "hold" on her blood pressure medication. ER took X-rays and did an MRI and discovered massive bruising in her hip area, but no fracture. Chest X-ray was okay. Reluctantly, we took her back to the home at 10:00 p.m. I had quite a talk with our favorite med aide. She revised her shift to be on duty at night to check on Penny. Between the three of us—Debbie, Michele, and myself— we were "looking over their shoulder" as many hours as we could. I slept, due to exhaustion, about four hours a day. We had the best doctor of our lives. What bothered me was knowing that many families do not have such a team. We had our doctor, our pharmacist, and Debbie with her medical knowledge, plus our network of medical professionals. How much longer would it be until our doctor demanded that we move Penny out of the glorified Taj Mahal? We were waiting for feedback from adult foster homes, trying to find a vacancy in a facility that provided level-3 care for Alzheimer's residents, plus an RN.

October 23. I visited and found her sleeping in a lounge chair. The med aide said she had a good rest and had taken her meds.

October 24. Michele and I visited with Murph, her terrier mix, who was happy to see Penny. After petting Murph, she was in good spirits and walked with a bit of help. I took some bottles of Gatorade for Penny. Their comment: "The more Gatorade she drinks, the more she pees." Damn.

October 25. Doctor received a call from a newly hired nurse at MemHome—Penny's wound is getting worse. I met another wound nurse from HC. Home Care Coordinator told our doctor that Penny's daughter was washing the wound—a damned lie. The bottles of Gatorade marked for Penny were gone. Their only excuse was, "Oh, we must have given them to someone else."

October 26. Medical aide took Penny's blood pressure at 7:00 a.m.—77/37. They began pushing fluids. At 1:30 p.m. it was 103/41; at 4:00 p.m., 110/60; at 7:00 p.m., 117/62.

October 27. I called the med aide at 7:30 a.m. to have them take her blood pressure before giving her meds. They said, "If it's low, our hands are tied." I called an MD at our doctor's clinic. He then called the Care Coordinator to withhold Penny's blood pressure meds. He was furious when we talked, saying, "Damn it, the medication is marked on the packaging label: Withhold medication if BP is below 90/60." Apparently, the med aides could not read and would not call the doctor. Instead, they kept giving her BP meds no matter how low it went. It was threatening her life. These idiots were flirting with disaster.

October 28. She had low blood pressure in the morning—82/48 and 81/44—no meds. They gave her more water. I called the doctor to see what BP level requires an IV. By then her blood pressure was 103/54. I left at 5:00 p.m. when the med aides assured me they would stay with her, pushing fluids and elevating her feet. Our special med aide took the next shift to ensure Penny received the attention required.

Great news: We finally received word that Penny was accepted at the new adult foster home a few minutes from our home and St. Vincent hospital. Thank you, Lord. On October 29, we moved Penny out of the glorified MemHome care facility in Oregon

City. I took her out the front entrance by the main dining room, the offices, and reception area. We made about five trips with her furniture and clothes. Not one person asked me what I was doing. I also noticed that aides were wearing jackets and sweaters that had been "lost" from Penny's closet. Most of her clothes had Nordstrom labels. She had just been subjected to a 60-Day Adventure in Hell. It was like a Sci-Fi TV series. Many of the people I've talked with over the years said their female friends who were admitted to a large memory care facility died within three months from urinary tract infections. Poor hygiene care?

CHAPTER 7

FINAL SEPARATION

October 29, 2012. Penny's new home in Northwest Portland was like a resort. It was very clean. She was the only resident with AD. It was a very nice facility with a country atmosphere. It was a converted five-bedroom home (sold for $800,000 in 2010). Owners/managers lived on the second level. Great caregivers from Mexico, Romania, and Ukraine.

October 30. I joined Penny for breakfast. Her blood pressure was 139/79 at 9:00 a.m. She was in good spirits, and watched deer playing in the field while eating. I left and came back at 1:30 p.m. She was napping in her room with a TV.

October 31. Doctor's appointment. Very pleased with her progress in such a short time.

November 1. Penny walked around the living room, and read the newspaper. Staff tried to keep her from sleeping. They said she was up until 3:00 a.m.

Week of November 4. Sunday. Improving each day. Ashley and Debbie visited. Penny recognized her great-grandson from photos. Strange how our brain can function better when it gets liquids.

Monday. Wound nurse visited. The wound was much better, getting smaller. Michele visited and put on TED hose.

Tuesday. Penny was in good spirits. She took her first shower in the huge, tiled Roman bathroom at 2:30 p.m. She did not like it. I screwed up and the water was not warm enough. Her blood pressure was 137/83. Aide put on TED hose in the morning.

Wednesday. Good spirits. She danced around living room. Her blood pressure was 124/71 at 10:00 a.m.

December 28. Took Penny to St. Vincent emergency room, where tests revealed problems with muscles, dehydration, and an urinary tract infection (UTI)—her second in a year. With each UTI, the AD stage advances a year or more. A typical bacteria count is 105–170. Hers was 170,000. On Sunday she recognized me as her father rather than husband, but she did recognize Debbie. Fed her breakfast, a tiny amount of applesauce and oatmeal. She sipped water through a straw. At the advice of two staff doctors at St. Vincent, I signed forms to start hospice for six months. If her condition improves, she can go off hospice. She ate very little for lunch—mashed potatoes with gravy, applesauce, sipped apple juice.

Monday. Checked out of St. Vincent and returned to foster home.

Tuesday. Penny ate a breakfast of eggs in her wheelchair. Michele noticed a lump in her left calf that was sore to the touch. Blood clot?

Note: Before Penny went on oxygen, Brix, the home's resident dog, howled and cried all night outside her room. As soon as she was placed on oxygen, Brix became quiet. Her heavy breathing alerted him.

Wednesday. Hospice nurse to visit and check lump. Hospice social worker gave Penny a shower.

Friday, January 4. We discussed memorial service with Pastor Lyda at St. Matthew Lutheran Church in Beaverton.

Saturday. Michele and I visited Pioneer Cemetery site in Naselle, Washington. Penny's temperature that evening was 102.

Sunday. Penny stopped eating. She couldn't swallow. She was taking no medications except Tylenol and morphine. Her temperature ranged from 101.7 to 99 by 7:00 p.m. Blood pressure 120/60, pulse 72 to 100 by 8:00 p.m. Breaths per minute (BPM) ranged from 16 to 20. Her temperature varied from 99.8 to 102.

Monday. Her pulse varied from 76 to 100.

Tuesday. Her temperature varied from 100.6 to 101.4; BPM was 14 to 20; pulse was 60 to 84. Blood pressure was 72/40. That night, at 11:00 p.m., Pastor Lyda was there for the Lutheran doxology and anointed her with oil. It was a very pleasant moment.

Wednesday. We were all there to see her take her last breath and squeeze our hands at 3:27 p.m. Pastor Lyda and the hospice chaplain visited the home. Hospice sent a lady to the home with a small harp to play and sing. It was very comforting knowing she will be in a better world. Thank you, Lord.

Penny's memorial service was exceptional. Mandy developed a full-color, four-page Celebration of Life program featuring her photo, A Life Remembered, a poem, "My Beloved Wife," that I wrote in basic training in 1953, and a photo of us holding hands at our 60th wedding anniversary.

The support of our pastor, family, friends, and medical people, plus my Lutheran faith, brought me through a very rough few years in my life.

Michele and I visited the Pioneer Cemetery near Naselle, Washington, to review the marble memorial marker. Our dogs Murph and Max accompanied us on our two-hour drive. It was a pleasant sunny day. The dogs had never visited this site. When the car turned off the county road to the cemetery driveway, the dogs began crying and whimpering as they peered out the windows. When we stood by the marker, both dogs began howling, with their noses in the air. They knew this was Penny's resting place, although this was their first visit. The wisdom of animals, our dogs.

ALZHEIMER'S DISEASE: WHAT ARE THE WARNING SIGNS?

We may think we are living and enjoying the good life, but there are hidden dangers we can avoid for ourselves and our loved ones. Look for the warning signs of Alzheimer's disease. Following are a few examples:

- Cannot follow numbered or logical sequence. In answering a Department of Motor Vehicles Driver's Test, rather than answering in order, 1 through 15, they work on #1, then skip to #7, back to #3, then #9 ... seldom completing all the answers.
- May have trouble cooking a meal and following the sequence of preparation through clean-up.
- May become confused about where kitchen items are stored. May put glassware with staples, towels with kettles.
- May write checks to pay utility bills more than once.
- May have problems balancing their checking account.
- Observe the person driving their car. If they seem confused, consult their doctor to request a driver's license examination from DMV. This procedure is less stressful than having a family member take away their keys.
- Observe the person while they are making out holiday or birthday greeting cards.
- Observe the person setting the thermostat in their home, if they have done so in the past.
- Observe the person compiling a grocery shopping list and filling it at the supermarket.

TAKE CONTROL

We are foolish to think there are those whose only interest is to ensure our health and well-being. There are situations that are intentional and unintentional that could put our health and well-being at risk. We do not invest blindly in our property, our materials, or our children's education. Wisely, we seek advice. Then why would we invest blindly in our health and well-being? Seek advice—a second, third opinion.

1. If your friend or relative seems to reveal the early signs of AD, ensure that their wealth is protected. It's best to take care of the bank accounts, investments, real estate, and will earlier rather than later in court. A hint to their attorney and banker could be in order.
2. If they practice in your area, seek out medical doctors who specialize in geriatrics and AD.
3. Seek out support groups through churches, medical centers, senior citizen groups, etc. You will burn yourself out navigating alone.

DEVELOP THE PROPER ATTITUDE

Your emotions must be controlled to ensure the benefits of improving your behavior in assisting your loved ones. As AD progresses, there will be times when it seems you are caring for a three-year-old, then a two-year-old and finally, a one-year-old child. If this is an avenue you are not prepared to travel, seek advice from your personal doctor. I had the ideal support team: our doctor (I went through three to find a great one; she was in her early thirties), our pastor, our pharmacist, our two daughters (one with a BS in Nursing), plus our extended family, friends, and relatives. During the late evenings when I was at my computer working on this book, I thought about the seniors who were alone or a couple, one with AD. I am blessed with an angel peering over my work, encouraging me.

CHAPTER 8

WHAT IS THIS DISEASE? THE INVESTIGATION OF ALZHEIMER'S DISEASE

"The scientist discovers the world that exists ... the engineer creates the world that never was."

–Theodore von Karman, PhD, a
Hungarian-American aerospace engineer and
physicist and consultant to Jack Northrop

Since I was a youngster, I have been fascinated with how mechanical things work. What makes them tick? My passion was disassembling old clocks—big clocks—and parts off old automobiles to see how they worked. How did a windshield wiper mechanism go one direction then the other? How do hydraulic brakes work? At the age of nine, I built my first bicycle from old parts found in a junkyard. I was an auto mechanic at 15. My 16-year-old buddy and I re-powered his 1931 Model A Ford roadster with a V-12 Lincoln engine complete with the steering column shifting linkage to the 1941 Lincoln side-shift transmission. Henry Ford was a genius—everything fit together.

Many years later, my passion led to an engineering degree. As a retired engineer, I donned my applied research hat to seek additional answers concerning health issues—HIV/AIDS, cancer, and heart disease in the 1980s, and Alzheimer's disease beginning in the mid-1990s. Let's call it my investigation of Alzheimer's disease. As the messenger, I'll wear two hats: engineer and investigative detective/reporter.

What factors contribute to Alzheimer's disease?

First, where is AD more likely to occur in the female population over 70 years of age? Maybe there's a correlation in the regions indicating diet, lifestyle, or whatever other reasons I can find under the rocks. I searched the internet and found the highest rate of dementia—Alzheimer's disease—was in England, Finland, and certain states in the United States, where it has doubled since 1980. Why Finland? Being Finnish and Swedish, I was quite concerned. My wife was half Swedish. One reason is because the soils in each country are depleted of selenium and other essential minerals. What about the other Scandinavian countries: Denmark, Norway, and Sweden? Why is Finland the only Scandinavian country with a high rate of AD? Actually, Finland has the highest death rate due to AD in the world. The US is in the top five. There is a simple explanation for an engineer—the glacial soils in Finland lack selenium. We don't need a $25 million grant with a 10-year study by a "politically savvy university" to confirm the findings.

In the United States, more than 45% of the general population over 85 has Alzheimer's disease. At 65, it is only 5%. People in Nigeria have rates as low as 1.4%, as does India. African Americans have rates of more than 6%. In rural Japan, the rate is near 4%. Japanese people living in Hawaii and the US have rates over 8%.

What is selenium?

Selenium is a trace mineral that is essential to good health. Selenium is incorporated into selenoproteins, which are antioxidant enzymes. They prevent cell damage caused by free radicals that may contribute to the development of chronic diseases such as Alzheimer's, cancer, cardiovascular disease, etc. Selenoproteins also help regulate the thyroid and contribute to the immune system.

What foods provide selenium?

Plant foods are the major dietary sources in the world. The selenium content in food depends on the content of selenium in the soil where the plants are grown or the animals are raised. Low-selenium soils are found in Eastern and Northern Europe, including Finland, which has glacial regions. Soils from the high plains of northern Nebraska and the Dakotas have high levels of selenium. Most of the Alaskan soils are selenium deficient. Regions of China and Russia have very low levels of selenium in their soils. Selenite, a selenium mineral, is added to table salt in regions of China as a requirement instituted by public health officials in 1991. (Understanding Selenium, by C. Leigh Broadhurst, Vitamin Retailer, September 2003.) Selenium can also be found in meats and seafood. In the US, meats (beef, turkey, chicken), seafood (cod, salmon, sardines, and tuna) and bread are common sources of dietary selenium. Brazil nuts contain very high levels of selenium—over 500 micrograms per ounce.

What is the recommended dietary allowance of selenium?

RDA for adults (19 years-plus) will range from 20 to 55 mcg with a maximum of 400 mcg. Excess amounts of selenium are a health risk. It is toxic in large amounts.

E. Will Taylor, PhD, a viral researcher at the University of Georgia-Athens, finds it intriguing that a number of viruses (Ebola,

HIV-1, etc.) have emerged from Zaire, Africa, an area where the soils appear to be selenium deficient. He theorized that several little-known genes in HIV control the formation of selenocysteines, proteins with a ravenous appetite for selenium. ("Selenium deficiency, Ebola, AIDS" by E. Will Taylor, PhD, 2005.)

Selenium deficiency may contribute to:

- AIDS/HIV
- Alzheimer's
- Arthritis
- Cancer—colorectal, lung, and prostate (selenium acts as an antioxidant, preventing/slowing tumor growth—studies performed as early as 1970)
- Cataracts
- Ebola
- Heart disease—cholesterol and high blood pressure
- Kashin-Beck disease, which results in osteoarthropathy

In 2009, the roof caved in on the supplement industry. Selenium was receiving too much attention in the media as a supplement that may reduce the risk of various chronic diseases (listed above). The Food and Drug Administration rode in on their white steed, wielding their mighty sword. Another Crusade? With adrenaline flowing, they were on the scene to defend the pharmaceutical industry (with a mere $300 billion in sales). There's no money in prevention. Herbs and minerals are not patentable. What if selenium supplements gained a foothold and reduced the numbers of people getting chronic diseases in the world? Heaven forbid. Big Pharma might see their revenues drop by a few percentage points. The FDA was on the scene to prevent such a disaster from occurring.

Keshan disease—a viral disease of the heart muscle—was discovered in China (Keshan County in Heilongjiang Province) in the 1930s. The disease peaked in the 1960s after claiming thousands of lives. It also is found in China's Yunnan Province, Finland, New Zealand, and Russia.

Further information on this subject can be found on various websites, including the Linus Pauling Institute, *The Nutrition Reporter*, and *Vitamin Retailer*. There also is data from studies in China, France, Japan, and the United States that were conducted in the 1980s and 1990s, and the website of the National Institutes of Health, with information from 2003 to the present.

Australia's Queensland Brain Institute reports that scientists believe selenium deficiency is how Ebola, HIV, and similar viruses become more powerful and develop resistance to drugs. A British researcher suggests low selenium levels may even be part of the reason Mad Cow disease spread so quickly throughout Europe.

Other co-risk factors that may contribute to Alzheimer's include ("It's Not Always Alzheimer's" by Elizabeth A. Reid, *Elks Magazine*, October 2007):

- Aluminum, fluoride, and lead absorption—a toxic trifecta
- Anti–
    » anxiety agents
    » depressants
    » histamines
    » Parkinsonian agents
    » spasmodics
    » psychotics

- Cardiac drugs (digoxin)
- Diuretics
- Pain relievers (opiates such as codeine, fentanyl, heroin, hydrocodone, methadone, morphine, naloxone, opioids, opium, oxycodone, Percodan, Vicodin)
- Sedatives

- Non-steroidal anti-inflammatory drugs (aspirin, ibuprofen, naproxen, and celecoxib)
- smoking

THE RELATIONSHIP OF ALUMINUM AND ALZHEIMER'S

On my patio, I have a cast aluminum planter for flowers and vegetables that is patterned after the 17th-century lead planters from a castle in France. Strange, but I have never been able to get flowers or leeks to grow and appear healthy in the planter. The same items planted in the same potting soil in a wood planter are healthier than those in the aluminum planter. If the aluminum has such a detrimental effect on flowers, it stands to reason that it would be harmful to the human body, but less noticeable. But to this day, we still find aluminum in our food products. Why? I'm waiting for an answer from the FDA and the USDA.

Virtually every research project associated with Alzheimer's disease has shown high concentrations of brain aluminum during an autopsy. People in every section of the United States are affected by toxic levels of aluminum—sometimes four to six times the amount found in the normal brain. ("It's Not Always Alzheimer's" by Elizabeth A. Reid, *Elks Magazine*, October 2007) This problem is becoming endemic across the land. The human body has no need for aluminum. Aluminum has no nutritional function. It aids no enzyme reactions. Aluminum accumulation in the body may lead to a number of health complications as we grow older. Aluminum is found in all types of consumer products associated with our body. We cook with aluminum cookware. We cover our food with aluminum foil (food changes before we ingest it when we cook in aluminum, and also when we use the convenient aluminum foil to cover our food). The mineral is found in buffered aspirin, antacids, and antiperspirants. Many currently used antiperspirants list aluminum zirconium tetrachlorohydrex gly as the active ingredient. To plug your pores, sweat glands? Aluminum salts are used in our drinking water systems for purification. Even non-alcoholic beverages contain aluminum. Aluminum is also found in IV solutions and a few baby formulas. Kidney dialysis patients are exposed to aluminum. We find it in non-dairy creamers, processed cheese, even hemorrhoid preparations. Adults can pass aluminum in their urine; infants do not have this ability. The levels of aluminum in infant formulas are higher than those in human milk. (Toxic chemicals in everyday products. *www.takepart.com/article/2013/10/28*). Why?

Here's a brief primer on elementary school chemistry: Aluminum comes from a clay-like substance called bauxite through the application of heat in aluminum reduction mills. History tells of aluminum being more valuable than gold dating back to the second century AD. Potash alum, which is derived through the leaching of alumina from bauxite, appears in Pliny's *Natural History*. (Pliny the Elder, ad 23–ad 79, was a natural historian who died during the eruption of Mount Vesuvius in Italy.) Potash alum (aluminum potassium sulfate) is used for water purification and in food preparation, pickling, etc. Soda alum (mendozite) is used for making baking powder. Ammonium alum (sulfate of aluminum) is used for water purification, vegetable glues, porcelain cements, deodorants, and dyeing and fireproofing textiles. Chrome alum (sulfate of chromium and potassium) is used in tanning leather. Selenate-containing alums contain selenium and are used as oxidizing agents. Aluminum sulfate (papermaker's alum) is used for industrial flocculation in the water purification process.

Dating as far back as 1885, aluminum has been considered the culprit in causing Alzheimer's. Tests revealed aluminum to be toxic to the nervous tissues of animals. ("Alzheimer's Again Linked to Aluminum" by Dr. John McDougall, McDougall Wellness Center, www.rense.com/general37/alum.htm) With aluminum being the third most common element on the planet's surface, we are exposed through numerous sources. Most of these sources are under our control. Since research and testing began to determine if aluminum was in fact the cause of Alzheimer's, the jury has been confused and frustrated. For eight years, from 1979 to 1987, there was a 1,300-percent increase in the number of deaths from Alzheimer's disease in the United States. ("Aluminum and Alzheimer's Disease: A New Look" by AC Miu, O Benga (Romania), *Journal of Alzheimer's Disease*, Vol. 10, #2, March 2006, 179-201. http://iospress.metapress.com)

To most of us, there is enough evidence to place the caution sign on aluminum. Avoid it if you can. Buy alternative products. By trying to "pinpoint" aluminum as the cause of Alzheimer's, the "political scientists" have laid a "smoke screen" for those of us who are not scientists or health professionals. By their use of the phrase "inconclusive as *the* cause," aluminum will remain in our water treatment plants, our food products, and other consumer items. Aluminum *is* a risk factor in Alzheimer's disease, along with numerous others.

The message between the lines of the complete article is that the involvement of aluminum in the pathogenesis of Alzheimer's disease should not be disregarded, especially in these times when those preaching the amyloid dogma of Alzheimer's etiology are demonstrating their myopia.

The aluminum cause-link to the Alzheimer's controversy has joined the ranks of other research projects. Rather than being "true science" they have entered a field that I dub "political science." Two scientific research programs in the Pacific Northwest, the Chinook (King) salmon and the Northern spotted owl, are examples of "political science" programs.

To date, the aluminum link to Alzheimer's controversy is alive and well. Since 1976, Dr. Henry Wisniewsky (1931–1999) was one of the most prominent scientists researching Alzheimer's. He was considered the most eminent neuroscientist of the twentieth century. At conferences he was one to challenge the linking of aluminum to Alzheimer's. The American Aluminum Association, based in Washington, DC, has a strong lobby group that challenges the link theory of aluminum to AD. They argue that the evidence is inconclusive. And from whom do you think Dr. Wisniewsky received his funding to continue his work? The American Aluminum Association. In 1988, the AAA helped him set up the Center for Trace-Element Studies, of which he was the director. (Aluminum and Alzheimer's, Celina Bell, February 22, 1996, www.cleanairpurewater.com/alum.html) Scientists with a "leaning" toward the AAA (aluminum industry) hesitate to tell the complete story. They rely on "... in disclosing the facts"—a neat trick in scientific journalism. Ellipses (...) denote a break or gap, where a part is missing or lost. Most of the time, the missing part can change the meaning of the statement. It's a form of wordsmithing.

A study conducted in Ontario, Canada, in the 1990s concluded that communities with high levels of aluminum in their drinking water had higher levels of Alzheimer's disease. (See Celina Bell article above) The water board in Sydney, Australia, hired a consultant to study whether alum could be absorbed by the body. In the study, the consultant gave rats Sydney tap water treated with alum. After two weeks, their brains were examined, and aluminum was present. This was the first study (1990s) that revealed a direct path from drinking water, across the gastrointestinal tract, into the bloodstream and then into the brain. The Sydney Water Board decided against the use of aluminum in their new water plant, the second largest in the world. (See Celina Bell article above) Although most of the funding and efforts pursue research into the genetic link, the latest research reveals that less than 1% of Alzheimer cases are inherited. (Controversial Claims About Causes of Alzheimer's Disease, June 16, 2009, www.webmd.com/alzheimers) Politically motivated "science"?

Aluminum has long been known as a neurotoxic agent. It is an etiopathogenic factor in diseases related to long-term dialysis treatment, and it has been controversially invoked as an aggravating factor or co-factor in Alzheimer's disease as well as in other neurodegenerative diseases. ("The role of metals in neurodegenerative processes: aluminum, manganese, and zinc" Paolo Zatta, et al, University of Padova, Italy, www.sciencedirect.com/science/science/article/pii)

In my opinion as an engineer, aluminum contributes to AD. By trying to label it as *the* cause, "political scientists" and the aluminum lobbyists are only exacerbating the controversy. I'm not waiting for the AAA, AMA, FDA, and our legislators to decide the correct action for my health and well-being. I'm still in control. After working in heavy industry (fabrication of various metals, casting, machining, welding) for more than 30 years, I had the taste of metals in my mouth. It was like putting my tongue on a clean plate of aluminum, brass, copper, iron, steel, etc. It became more noticeable while I was taking a hot shower. Being one who believes in cleansing our body by herbs, minerals, and vitamins, I took a cleanse regime (one packet of a formulation of twenty-three herbs and vitamins) with a large glass of water twice a day for a month. The all-natural products worked in harmony with my body to cleanse my digestive system, liver, kidneys, and blood to the point where I no longer could taste metals. That was over 40 years ago. I continue a cleanse regimen monthly with a cleanse tea for two weeks. Lemon juice is also a good detox item. The latest trendy detox drink is celery juice.

OTHER FACTORS AND THEORIES

My investigation of aluminum crossed paths with the fluoridation of our water. Fluoride (sodium fluoride) is a toxic by-product of industry, one being aluminum reduction mills. As such, alum (aluminum sulfate) and sodium fluoride are partners in crime.

They combine in our blood to form aluminum fluoride, which *does* pass through the blood-brain barrier. Aluminum fluoride is poisonous to our kidneys. Aluminum salts in the brain lead to Alzheimer's. Together in our water systems, they add another co-risk factor for Alzheimer's (*Journal of the American Medical Association*; Dr. S.J. Jacobsen, 1990; C. Danielson, 1992; Medical Research Endocrinology Dept.; England; University of Ruhana, Sri Lanka; *Journal of the National Academy of Research Biochemists*, Jan/Feb 1990; Brain Research, vol. 784– 1998; Senior Research Scientist, MIT; Senior Scientist, US Navy).

If the addition of lead is found in our body, a "trifecta" exists. The combination of aluminum, fluoride, and lead results in a more severe toxin. This is attributed to a synergistic process. Canada, Cuba, Finland, Germany, the Netherlands, and North Carolina report additional studies. There are more than nine million sites on the internet devoted to Alzheimer's connection to fluoridation. As my investigation revealed, there are more than fifty co-risk factors for Alzheimer's. In my profile of AD patients (friends and family) there was a group of risk factors that, combined, contribute to the disease—perhaps as many as eight or more. Depending upon the concentration of the co-risk factors, the disease will develop.

Dr. Klinghardt explains his 9 Steps to Detox in "The Klinghardt Neurotoxin Elimination Protocol," where he addresses neurotoxins such as heavy metals—mercury, lead, cadmium, and aluminum; biotoxins; xenobiotics; food preservatives, etc. (The Klinghardt Neurotoxin Elimination Protocol, Dietrich Klinghardt, MD, PhD, American Academy of Neural Therapy, Bellevue, WA., Academies in UK, Germany, Switzerland. www. hbci.com/wenonah/new/9steps/htm)

Medical books from the 1970s written by Paavo Airola, ND, PhD, stressed the lemon juice cleanse to rid our bodies of chemicals. Mix the juice of ten lemons in two quarts of water and sweeten with honey. Drink one glass every two hours. It cleanses the liver. Dr. Airola suggests the lemon cleanse be done a few times a year. Dr. Airola (1918–1983) studied biochemistry, nutrition, and natural healing in medical centers in Germany, Sweden, and Switzerland. He was a visiting lecturer at Stanford University Medical School.

Forty years later, the lemon cleanse is being promoted by the Institute of Health Sciences of Baltimore, MD. However, they have added another benefit: lemon (citrus) is a miraculous product to kill cancer cells. They claim it destroys the malignant cells in twelve types of cancers, including breast, colon, lung, pancreas and prostate.

When I googled "Institute of Health Sciences" a site of Health Sciences Institute appeared with their mission: "Dedicated to uncovering and researching the most urgent advances in modern underground medicine."

Dr. James Lind (1716–1794) from England discovered the cause and prevention of scurvy: a lack of vitamin C from citrus such as lemons. Scurvy patients lack collagen, the stuff that holds our tissues together. Without collagen, Dr. Lind found that patients would bleed and bruise easily, and ultimately their hearts would fall apart. Thanks to the culprit of bureaucracy, it took the British Navy 50 years to implement Dr. Lind's findings. It took the American Navy 75 years to accept his findings.

Dr. Cal McCausland, Chief Scientific Officer at 4Life Research, (PhD, organic chemistry), considers Vitamin C to be the link to lifetime health and wellness. He is the first American to receive a membership and the title of Academician in the Russian Federation Academy of Medical Technical Sciences (equivalent to Knighthood in England).

Dr. Linus Pauling (1901–1994) was the only person to be awarded two unshared Nobel Prizes, in Chemistry and Peace. He was among the first scientists to work in the fields of quantum chemistry and molecular biology, earning a PhD in physical chemistry and mathematical physics from the California Institute of Technology. There were times when Dr. Pauling was ridiculed for his claims about Vitamin C. Learned medical doctors stated he should be placed in a straitjacket. At one time, the medical establishment considered Dr. Pauling to be a quack. The American Medical Association and the USFDA did not want to embrace Dr. Pauling's findings. Dr. Pauling lived into his nineties.

Certain diseases of memory, like Wernicke-Korsakoff psychosis, revealed in thiamine or vitamin B_1 deficiency can strikingly impair the ability to make new memories. This results in the patient living in the past, with new memories lost forever. This condition is common with alcoholics and malnourished people. A few patients display Transient Global Amnesia from lack of blood supply to the brain, which causes a temporary inability to make new memories for minutes or hours, though behavior is normal. Fugue state, a rare psychiatric disorder in patients with Psychiatric Dissociative States or Temporal Lobe Epilepsy, can produce unplanned travel/ wandering along with poor memory recall and formation.

In 2007, a professor from Northwestern University theorized that immunotherapy and specific antibodies that target beta-amyloid protein could reverse Alzheimer's if caught in the early stages. These early stage beta-amyloid toxins, called oligomers, make it impossible for people to form new memories. The research suggested that Alzheimer's may be a type of immune deficiency disorder. The director of the Mayo Clinic's Alzheimer's disease center considers the research credible. Oligomers disrupt memory at very low concentrations and can cause brain cell death, according to the director of the Memory Disorders Program at New York-Presbyterian/Weill Cornell Medical Center.

In 2008, a research team at the Klein Lab disclosed their years of research describing Alzheimer's disease as a form of diabetes. They have shown that a toxic protein called ADDL in the brains of people with Alzheimer's removes insulin receptors from nerve cells, rendering those neurons insulin resistant. "We think this is a major factor in the memory deficiencies caused by ADDLs in Alzheimer's brains," said Dr. William Klein, a member of Northwestern's Cognitive Neurology and Alzheimer's Disease Center. (About Alzheimer's, www.kleinlab.org/aboutalzheimers.htm, Discovery Supports Theory of Alzheimer's Disease as Form of Diabetes, www.research.northwestern.edu/news/stories/2008/klein.html)

Homocysteine is no doubt a new word for many of you readers. I was introduced to homocysteine more than 25 years ago while reading about Kilmer S. McCully, MD. Dr. McCully was engaged in heart research at Harvard University. He had an unusual article published in the *American Journal of Pathology*. His article revealed the possibility of an entirely new cause of heart disease. Dr. McCully found that children with elevated levels of homocysteine showed signs of blood vessel degeneration similar to those of adults with heart disease. Rather than being rewarded for this new finding, Harvard handed the gifted research scientist his pink slip. Fellow scientists denounced him, others ignored him. Why was his research scorned by his medical colleagues? Professional jealousy? You can take that to the bank.

His research grants ceased. He remained active by taking a job in pathology at a veterans hospital. Years later, heart researchers and scientists around the globe were embracing his findings, as did Harvard, finally. ("The Fall and Rise of Kilmer McCully" by Michelle Stacey. *New York Times Magazine*, Aug. 10, 1997.) *T Journal of American Medical Association* reviewed 209 studies lin homocysteine with heart disease (HOMOCYSTEINE: The Cause of Heart Disease?). Dr. McCully discovered that homocysteine levels could be reduced with supplem vitamin B_6, folic acid, and vitamin B_{12}, rather tha therapy. Heaven forbid.

Elevated homocysteine levels are asso

health conditions, including Alzheimer's disease, birth defects (neural tube), cardiovascular disease, depression, diabetes, multiple sclerosis, osteoporosis, and rheumatoid arthritis. Current research indicates that homocysteine should be considered a co-risk factor for AD. The full article, by Dr. W. Arthur, cites twenty references dating back to 1975. ("Elevated Homocysteine Linked to Many Diseases" by W. Arthur, *Vitamin Retailer*, March 2006.)

Brain damage can occur during heart-bypass surgery. In most cases the cardiologist does not mention to their patient that one complication could be memory loss. This is but one of a series of side effects that can occur during heart-bypass surgery. These side effects of brain problems have been reported in medical journals since 1969. The *New England Journal of Medicine* reported in 2001 that five years after heart-bypass surgery, more than 40% of patients experienced a decline in their mental function. (Bill Clinton's Madness: A Consequence of Heart-Bypass Surgery Brain Damage. www.drmcdougal.com/misc/2008other/080412clinton.)

Clioquinol is an antifungal and antiprotozoal drug. In large doses the drug is neurotoxic (http://en.wikipedia.org.wiki//Clioquinol). The use of Clioquinol in both treatment and prevention of shigella infection was described in a report in 1964. The drug has been restricted or discontinued in some countries as the result of a problem in Japan between 1957 and 1970. Phase II clinical trials indicate that Clioquinol could halt cognitive decline
disease due to its ability to act as a chelator for
ons. Animal studies have shown that the drug
ression of Alzheimer's. The report warned
enting with this drug.
eview: Metal protein attenuating com-
atment of Alzheimer's disease (www.
5380.html). Summary: There is no
at has undergone a randomized
of 36 weeks is of benefit in

Alzheimer's disease. How long did it take the human body to show signs of Alzheimer's? Decades? Maybe the clinical trials should have continued for a couple years or more.

For more than 10 years, Ladostigil (TV-3,326) has been investigated for the treatment of neurodegenerative disorders such as Alzheimer's, Lewy body disease, and Parkinson's disease. Ladostigil combines the actions of the older drugs like rivastigmine and rasagiline into a single molecule. It also improves the expression of glial cell–derived neurotropic factor (GDNF) and brain-derived neurotropic factor (BDNF), and may be capable of reversing the damage caused by these diseases. GDNF was introduced as an experimental drug for Parkinson's by the manufacturer Amgen, Inc. They later withdrew the drug due to patient risks. Although many Parkinson's patients wanted the drug as their last ray of hope, the legal battle ended in favor of Amgen.

Artificial sweeteners have been around for years. When my father was taking insulin injections for diabetes (1943–1964), we kept saccharine in the cupboard for his use. However, one artificial sweetener in particular has been in the eye of the media and the consumer since it came out in the early 1980s. According to the numerous studies on aspartame, it contains chemicals that can have harmful effects in the human body, such as neurotoxic, metabolic, allergenic, fetal, and carcinogenic.

"We had better be sure that the questions that have been raised about the safety of this product are answered. I must say at the outset, this product was approved by the FDA in circumstances that can only be described as troubling," Ohio Sen. Howard Metzenbaum testified in a 1985 US Senate hearing on aspartame. The majority of the complaints volunteered to the FDA by customers concerned supplements that included aspartame. By 1995, the FDA had received more than 7,000 complaints. Alzheimer's disease has been associated with aspartame.

(Google: Aspartame Disease: An FDA-Approved Epidemic, by H.J. Roberts, MD.)

To the consumer (caregiver and patient), the controversy continues in the statin drug debate. If a person has Alzheimer's as well as high cholesterol, should they take statin drugs (Lipitor, Zocor, Mevacor, Pravachol, Crestor, Baycol, and others)? There are medical doctors and research scientists with clinical trials and studies that support each side of the fence with statin drugs.

During mid-year in 2001, my wife received a prescription for Baycol from her doctor to reduce her high cholesterol, which was near 300. I checked out the side effects of Baycol and hesitated to have her prescription filled. A few days later, the doctor said that Baycol had been recalled. She advised her not to take the medication. When my wife had heart-bypass surgery due to a blood clot 12 years before, she had many blood tests. The doctors were amazed. Although she had high cholesterol, they could not detect any plaque build-up in her blood vessels. Engineers would call this "impurities held in suspension"—as in automatic transmission fluid. The plaque was not "building-up" on the walls of her vessels. It was "floating" in the bloodstream where it would cause less damage, if any.

In 2000, research on statins, cholesterol-lowering drugs used to prevent heart disease and stroke, showed they may also reduce the risk of Alzheimer's disease. (Google: Cholesterol-Lowering Drug Reduces Dementia Risk by 70%—WebMD; Statins Fight Alzheimer's disease—WebMD; Cholesterol Drugs May Slow Alzheimer's—WebMD.) A recent study suggests people using the statin medications may be 70% less likely to get Alzheimer's disease and other dementia. In 2003, new research confirmed that cholesterol-lowering statin drugs could help prevent Alzheimer's disease. The preliminary findings appeared in the April issue of *Archives of Neurology*. Later, in 2005, French researchers reported slower mental decline in Alzheimer's patients who were taking cholesterol-lowering drugs. The study appeared in the *Journal of Neurology, Neurosurgery and Psychiatry*. The researchers at University Hospital in Lille, France, included Florence Pasquier, MD, PhD. They studied 342 Alzheimer's patients for about three years.

Side effects and drug toxicities from prescription medication take quite a toll on the consumer, as reported by the American Medical Association as well as studies by Johns Hopkins and Harvard Medical Universities. The term used is ADR—adverse drug reaction—which is responsible for more than 200,000 US deaths per year. Many older adults have been prescribed statin drugs to reduce their high cholesterol. While previous studies revealed a decreased risk of Alzheimer's with statin drugs, there are reports that statin drugs actually impair cognition. Recent studies with large numbers of subjects taking statin medications compared with a placebo group indicated no difference in cognition. Because statin drugs prevent the body from making CoQ10, which creates 95% of the body's energy, consumers should consider CoQ10 supplements to prevent depletion and reduction of oxidative stress on the brain.

Acetyl-l-carnitine acts as a powerful antioxidant that helps prevent brain cell deterioration. It also has been shown to improve insulin response. The body can make small amounts of l-carnitine, but requires multiple co-factors including vitamin C, B_6, niacin, iron, plus the amino acids lysine and methionine. Beef, lamb, and venison are good food sources of l-carnitine. The older adults who limit their diet of this nutrition to produce l-carnitine have another co-risk factor for cognitive decline.

The December 5, 2003, issue of *Share the Wealth* by Chris Gupta reveals stories concerning statin drugs and memory loss. (Google: Statin Drugs and Memory Loss.) Duane Graveline, MD, former NASA astronaut, USAF Flight Surgeon, Space Medicine Researcher and family doctor from Florida, tells of Transient

Global Amnesia, a side effect of statin drugs. (Google: "Statins: Are These Cholesterol-Lowering Drugs Right for You?" Mayo Clinic.)

Following are excerpts from a four-page article written by Mayo Clinic staff and posted on the internet:

"Should you be on statins? These cholesterol-lowering drugs have benefits and risks. Find out whether your risk factors for heart disease make you a good candidate for statin therapy. Statins include well-known medications such as Lipitor, Zocor, Mevacor, Pravachol, Crestor and others. High cholesterol means your total cholesterol level is 240 mg/dl or higher—or, your 'bad cholesterol' (LDL) level is 130 mg/dl or higher. Risk factors for heart disease include high cholesterol, family history, inactive lifestyle, high blood pressure, age, poor health, having diabetes, overweight, smoking, or having peripheral artery disease. If your only risk factor is high cholesterol, you may not need the statin drugs. The side effects of statin drugs include muscle and joint aches, nausea, diarrhea, constipation. The more serious side effects include liver damage and muscle problems." Note: The Mayo report did not mention potential memory loss (Kukull, Walter A., et al., Solvent Exposure as a Risk for Alzheimer's Disease: A Case-Control Study, *American Journal of Epidemiology*, 1995, 141:1059-71).

A potent anti-tumor necrosis factor alpha treatment was approved for rheumatoid arthritis in 1997. A method of treating TNF-dependent inflammatory diseases in a mammal by administering a TNF antagonist, such as soluble TNFR, was invented and patented by C.A. Jacobs and C.A. Smith, who assigned their invention to Immunex Corporation in Seattle. A short time later, Edward Tobinick, MD, patented (US #6,015,557 and others) "The Tobinick Method" of off-label treatment of selected patients with Alzheimer's disease. Dr. Tobinick is an assistant clinical professor of medicine at UCLA and director of the Institute for Neurological Research in Los Angeles. (Google: Dr. Edward Tobinick, MD)

Note the players in the etanercept product:

- Inventors: C.A. Jacobs and C.A. Smith
- Product: A method of treating TNF-dependent inflammatory diseases in a mammal by administering a TNF antagonist, such as soluble TNFR.
- Assignee: Immunex Corporation, Seattle.
- The technology was acquired by Amgen in 2002.

Etanercept is co-marketed by Amgen and Pfizer under the trade name Enbrel in a powder form and a pre-mixed liquid. Wyeth markets Enbrel outside North America excluding Japan, where Takeda Pharmaceutical markets the drug.

The FDA approved etanercept for trauma, injury, and a number of neurological disorders, but not those associated with Alzheimer's disease.

Enbrel sales are in the $4–5 billion range annually—very successful for the manufacturer, Amgen, without any sales as a drug for AD treatment.

Dr. Edward Tobinick entered the scene with his development and patent (#6,015,557) for the "Repurposing of Enbrel for Alzheimer's Disease." This is termed "off-labeling" in the industry. If a product is approved by the FDA for one treatment and used for another, non-approved treatment, it is termed off-labeling. A host of new scientific "players and supporters" include the Institute of Neurological Research, University of Gothenburg (Gothenburg, Sweden); UC-Davis; University of Washington; Stanford; Northwestern; National Institute of Aging; Hotchkiss Brain Institute in Calgary (Alberta, Canada), and Trinity College Institute of Neuroscience in Dublin (Ireland).

Articles in medical journals with headlines reading "Reversal of Alzheimer's Symptoms Within Minutes in Human Study" spiked interest around the world. Would the anti-inflammatory drug etanercept help Alzheimer's patients? Dr. Tobinick co-authored a report documenting the fast improvement in a patient with Alzheimer's disease following administration of etanercept. ("Reversal of Alzheimer's Symptoms Within Minutes in Human Study" (sciencedaily.com, January 9, 2008))

In January of 2011, Wyeth and the University of Southampton began enrollment of a clinical trial of etanercept for patients with Alzheimer's.

The latest gossip on the internet indicates US physicians are offering to administer the off-label etanercept for treatment of Alzheimer's at a cost ranging from $40,000 to $100,000 annually.

"Political science" is raising its head in the use of etanercept treatments for Alzheimer's. When the patent expired in October 2012, it was unlikely that a generic would be available at that time—or ever. The United States is the only country that does not permit the manufacture of generic biologic drugs. A bill to change this situation has been stalled in the House Judiciary Committee. If a generic was allowed to be manufactured, the price would be greatly reduced.

What is the current status of clinical trials of etanercept (Enbrel) for Alzheimer's patients? I tried to find out the open trials and new trials as listed in the website of the National Institute on Aging in the US National Institutes of Health. Only one study is listed for etanercept: Enbrel and Alzheimer's. The Wyeth and University of Southampton (UK) study is in a holding pattern.

FYI, it's common knowledge in the pharmaceutical industry that the expense to advertise their drugs exceeds the cost to develop them. Industry people tell us a new drug will cost $350 million to $1 billion before it is released by the FDA and ready for the mass market, whereas "outsiders" claim the cost is more likely to range from $100 to $200 million. In the case of etanercept, it was developed by Immunex and sold to Amgen (Amgen bought Immunex for $10 billion). As for the use in patients with

Alzheimer's, the inventors did not start from a clean sheet of paper. They started with an FDA-approved anti-inflammatory drug.

Cogane is another promising drug for Parkinson's and Alzheimer's that went begging for clinical trial funds for five years. A foundation started by actor Michael J. Fox, himself a Parkinson's patient, gave the Phytopharm study a grant of $1.16 million. They were the darling on the London stock exchange while developing a drug based on plants for Alzheimer's. After reporting disappointing (to the investors) results from trials of its Alzheimer's treatment, their stock dropped 30%. The Emeritus Professor of Pharmacology at Oxford University who led the trials was surprised at the encouraging results.

After reading about the company and their trial it seemed like the investor crowd was impatient, wanting to achieve quick results. Their 90-day trial was promising, but not what the investors anticipated. The small research firm tabled their Alzheimer's drug and concentrated on Parkinson's. They did not have the funds to conduct their own larger, longer trial of Cogane for Alzheimer's. So, their clinical trials for Alzheimer's go begging for funding. Why?

Dr. Nicholas L. Meyers, PhD, Head of Development and Scientific Licensing at Phytopharm, replied to my email and gave me a review of their company. They have close collaboration with charitable organizations and leading scientists and clinicians to help guide the company's research and development activities.

In pre-clinical models of their administration of Cogane in conjunction with L-dopa, there was improved control of symptoms compared to being treated with L-dopa alone. The side effects of L-dopa were reduced. This data was presented at the International Congress of Parkinson's Disease and Movement Disorders in June of 2011, in Toronto, Canada.

Cogane was evaluated in a 400-patient multi-national Phase II, randomized, double-blind, placebo controlled, dose ranging study.

The study compared the safety, tolerability, and efficacy of three doses of Cogane and placebo when administered for 28 weeks to untreated patients with early stage Parkinson's disease. The study found no benefits. (Google: Phytopharm.com/research/cogane)

After considerable investigation, I became very alarmed. The majority of the risk factors that expose our bodies to Alzheimer's are out of our control.

Alarmed? Hell, I'm furious!

I found that the food we consume, the water we drink, the medicine we take, our work environment, and the air we breathe contribute to the co-risk factors in determining our likelihood of becoming a victim of Alzheimer's. By accident I found a link to another co-risk factor for Alzheimer's—solvents. They have been added as another co-risk factor. That's right—our adhesives, alcohols, benzene, ketones, paints, phenols, toluene, xylene (the list seems endless) contribute to our risk. They're not in the same category of risk factors as an AIDS victim having unprotected sex because that is their choice, and they are in control.

A study from 1987 to 1992 of about 23,000 people age 60 or over from an HMO in Seattle revealed that past exposure to organic solvents may be associated with onset of Alzheimer's disease. A painter in his late 50s had been exposed to various solvents for more than 30 years. The family and patient noticed impaired short-term memory function in his early 40s. (Google: Painter exposed to mixed solvents.)

Fresca is a soft drink produced by the Coca Cola Company. One of its ingredients is phenylketonurics, which contain phenylalanine (also found in eggs, milk, bananas, meat) and is 50% aspartame. Phenylalanine is a hidden danger to anyone consuming aspartame, an artificial sweetener that is an ester of methanol.

In 1996, the World Health Organization found that xylene's health effects caused damage to the nervous system. Xylene gets into drinking water mainly by the discharge from petroleum and chemical plants. Traces have been found in drinking water and tap water in New Orleans. Xylene can be introduced into our atmosphere by forest fires. A few controlled studies dating back to 1958 appear on the internet.

It was common during the 1940s and 1950s to wash the oil, grease, and grime off automobile parts using fire extinguisher fluid—carbon tetrachloride. Carbon tet was the best solvent to remove road tar from paint on an automobile. As a teenager, I had my hands and arms up to my elbows in a five-gallon container of carbon tet. Afterwards, I washed my hands and arms with waterless soap that included a lotion. Years later carbon tet was classified as highly carcinogenic.

A friend of mine served in the US Army at a major vehicle repair center in Germany. He said it was customary in the 1960s to wash the grime and carbon off of fuel system parts (jeeps to tank engines) with acetone, the nail polish remover, without masks and with no ventilation.

Inflammation may be a main contributor to our co-risk factors for Alzheimer's. I doubt if researchers will ever find one single cause of Alzheimer's.

What is clear is that Alzheimer's develops as a result of a complex cascade of biological processes that take place over many years inside the brain.

From the hundreds of reports I have reviewed, research has shown that numerous risk factors contribute to AD. The majority of research studies reveal that inflammation is linked to these risk factors.

The updates from 2005 to 2015 include the following contributors to inflammation:

- poor sleep quality
- low IQ
- the gum disease periodontitis

- social stresses such as feeling rejected
- overactive bladder
- types of meals
- unbalanced diet of omega-3 and omega-6
- low vitamin C
- high glycemic diet
- obesity
- diabetes
- post-traumatic stress disorder
- hostility and anger
- low carb diet
- depression
- Atkins diet
- job stress ... and more

Inflammation is also a contributor to arthritis, cancer, diabetes, enlarged prostate, heart disease, joint replacement, and vision loss. For detailed information on these inflammation studies, check out the source (http://inflammationfactor.com/research.php).

Although, inflammation is a natural healing body function, it can become a health problem when it is out of control.

Infections have become the latest culprit to raise havoc with an Alzheimer patient's brain. A mild infection can advance their memory decline by a year or more. The decline will be permanent, not temporary. Common infections among female AD patients are urinary tract infections. As I mentioned earlier, a friend of mine mentioned that three of her elderly lady friends, all Alzheimer's patients, died within three months of being admitted to an AD care facility. All had serious UTIs. This is common among female patients in facilities that provide poor hygiene care.

Dr. Oz (from TV) claims there are seven million UTIs a year in the US. Here is his list to reduce UTI's: maintain proper hygiene; drink eight glasses of water a day; drink prune juice and apple cider vinegar; eat avocados, nut butter, and seeds; change pads often, and avoid spicy foods, as they can aggravate a UTI.

When was the last time you observed a "Hazardous to Your Health" sign:

- ... on aluminum cookware, or foil?
- ... on your tap water, noted on your water bill?
- ... in your office, posted on every electronic device?
- ... on your prescription medication, other than side effects?

I could proceed, but I hope you see my point in trying to alarm you.

What will it take to alter your lifestyle so that *you* are in control?

- We consume drugs/medication like candy.
- We consume junk food as if it's our last supper.
- We smoke cigarettes, knowing we may die of cancer.
- We are overweight, praying for that magic pill or exercise DVD.
- We can't consume liquor in moderation; we need one more for the road.

We have become a nation of "overs"—over-indulgers, over-eaters, over-boozers, over-druggies, etc. We can be thankful for another group of "overs"—the overachievers who earn degrees in medicine and science who keep us from kicking the bucket at the ripe old age of 39.

All is not lost. If you've celebrated your 80th birthday, unless you smoked all your life, wolfed down "gut-bombs" with greasy fries from the roach coach for lunch every day, indulged in a few belts of booze every evening, retired as a painter, whatever you're doing, you'll likely see 85. For the rest of us, it's time to take control of what life we have remaining on this earth. For the over-indulgers, it's time to change.

Don't expect to abuse your body with booze, street drugs, junk food, and a detrimental lifestyle without consequences. The government may not offer to take care of your self-abused body. We're running out of money. On the current track our nation is traveling, AIDS, Alzheimer's, cancer, diabetes, and heart disease will run the money-well dry. I doubt if any politician will vote for another entitlement program allowing your self-abused body to die of old age.

My son-in-law shared some interesting articles on Alzheimer's. The two- and seven-page articles cited information from Dr. Richard Veech in Oxford, England; Dr. Wesley Thevathasan at John Radcliffe Hospital; Dr. David Diamond, Director of the Neuroscience Collaborative at University of South Florida; Dr. Suzanne de la Monte; and the blogs from Dr. Mary T. Newport.

In 2006, Dr. Andrew Dillin of the Salk Institute of Biological Studies in California, along with a team from Scripps Health, revealed their promising findings. They researched molecular janitors that clear away brain gunk—beta amyloid, and proteins HSF-1 and DAF-16. As of 2008, Andrew Dillin, a PhD in molecular and cellular biology, was a scientist at the Howard Hughes Medical Institute continuing his research of Alzheimer's. He currently runs a similar lab at the University of California, Berkeley.

CHAPTER 9

OUR RISK FACTORS
(co-risk factors, contributing factors)

Our investigation and research of Alzheimer's disease is incomplete. Further investigation and research will continue through our worldwide sources for future editions, as well as an AD blog. Alzheimer's is the most feared disease among adults polled, more than AIDS, cancer, and heart disease.

As of January 2011, our nation finally made research on Alzheimer's disease a high priority. The US was not the leader. The federal budget for Alzheimer's research for FY 2014 and 2015 was $115 million, while research for AIDS was $3 billion. Alzheimer's research has been a national priority in Australia, France, and the UK for many years. Dementia costs the UK economy 23 billion pounds yearly, more than cancer and heart disease combined.

Big Pharma has been burning the midnight oil trying to develop a drug that would treat, reverse and/or cure AD. After testing approximately 250 potential drugs, *not one* has passed Phase III Clinical Trials, which would allow the Food and Drug Administration to give the green light for marketing. Since the late 1990s, the cost for their efforts in developing AD drugs has been estimated at more than $800 billion. Note: The current drugs for Alzheimer patients were not developed by Big Pharma, but by foreign medical research groups. Pfizer Pharmaceutical has "thrown in the towel" on AD research, and others are following. While there are people who wish to wait for drugs from Big Pharma, those of us who embrace alternative, natural medicine, supplements, and a change in lifestyle can continue our path to health and well-being, while hoping others will follow.

My arthritis is controlled by supplements. I take one of the top anti-inflammation products on the market. Now that research has shown that inflammation is a co-risk factor in developing Alzheimer's, this product may be another hope and blessing for Alzheimer's patients wishing to take natural products rather than wait for the more expensive drugs with their inherent side effects.

As Hippocrates, the "Father of Medicine" (460–377 bc) so aptly expressed:

"Let thy food be thy medicine and let thy medicine be thy food."

Since around 2017 we have seen numerous television solicitations from law firms in regard to class action lawsuits concerning drugs. To name a few, there is Levaquin approved in 2003, with severe side effects involving tendon problems; as well as Celexa, Depakote, Effexor, Lexapro (approved in 2009), Paxil, Pristiq, Prozac (approved in 1987), Topamax, and Zoloft (approved in 1991), all of which have serious side effects including birth defects. Where Prozac is the drug of choice for depression here in the US, St. John's wort is the herb of choice in Europe for depression. The only publication I could find concerning the risk of drug interaction with St. John's wort was the FDA Public Health Advisory dated February 10, 2000. This related to St. John's wort and Indinavir for treating HIV. Although *Parade Magazine*, May 29, 2000 stated there was a list of 50 drugs that interact with St. John's wort, *no such list exists*, according to the FDA. The "pawns" of Big Pharma will go to any extreme to discredit St. John's wort. This popular herbal product has been prescribed internationally for the treatment of mild to moderate depression. I find it difficult to understand why the National Center for Complementary and Alternative Medicine, National Institute of Mental Health and the Office of Dietary Supplements would fund a multimillion dollar study to show that St. John's wort is ineffective for major depression.

Or, why would a study of St. John's wort be conducted by a group for digestive diseases at the Mayo Clinic that had set out to prove that St. John's wort does not ease irritable bowel syndrome? Yes, that was an actual study that tracked 70 patients from 2006 to 2008. It's okay with me if medical research groups have excess time and funds to conduct these studies, but I hope they don't use taxpayer money and that it's not to discredit a competing product. For years I have followed the "political science" of supplements vs. drugs in the *Journal of the American Medical Association, New England Journal of Medicine, Wall Street Journal, BusinessWeek, Time,* etc.

It seems as if the American Medical Association, the US Food and Drug Administration, and Big Pharma consider the supplement industry a thorn in their side. Since the beginning of recorded history there has always been a feud between physicians and herbal healers/medicine men/Salem witches. There are unsavory characters in each sector, charlatans, quacks, and snake oil peddlers. With over 50% of adults in the United States consuming supplements in a $40 billion market, the "Big Three"—Big Pharma, AMA, and FDA—do not want the supplement industry to grab a bigger piece of the healthcare pie. Where the supplement sector promotes prevention, the Big Three promote treatment. To create a healthy world at minimal cost, there must be a balance. In 2014, global medicinal drug sales totaled $1.1 trillion, including sales in the US of $330 billion. That's slightly less than US weapons sales by the Pentagon. There are big bucks in the treatment of disease, but very little in prevention.

My daughter brought me up to speed on a very promising treatment for breast cancer, possibly a cure. She was a director for a nonprofit group involved in medical research. Two medical doctors working independently on a cure for breast cancer were seeking the "missing link." One doctor was in need of A. The other doctor was in need of B. One doctor was at Harvard Medical Center and the other was at the small nonprofit group. They met through networking and discovered together that they had A and B. That was a few years ago. They are still in need of grant funding to conduct clinical trials. Are the investing community and our government so skewed that they will only consider funding research from the Fortune 500 giants and their associates? How do we prevent this form of infection from polluting our health and medical industries? *Or do we even care?*

My investigation into the contributing co-risk factors of Alzheimer's disease was quite alarming. Those victims of AD did not get the disease over a short period of time. For the co-risk factors to develop, it took many years, up to 30 or more. It is reasonable to surmise that stopping or possibly reversing the progression of AD also will take a long time.

Some of the drugs listed in the class action lawsuits took years to inflict their damage. Sometimes their damage was done during one pregnancy. Two of the drugs were approved by the FDA in 1987 and 1991. That's over 25 years ago. For a real eye-opener on how "political tactics" are utilized by various groups to shield a dangerous drug cocktail, one must peruse Alicia Mundy's words in *Dispensing with the Truth*. The battle over fen-phen brought my passion to a rolling boil. If I could go back 30 years in time, I would have returned to a university to earn a law degree. I do hope this ignites your passion for drugs vs. supplement knowledge. The separate drugs that became known as fen and phen had been on the market since the 1970s. In 1992 the "cocktail" of fen-phen was being promoted as a weight loss combo. They were a market success as a combo. During 1996 there were 18 million prescriptions being written each month. It was quite a money-maker. An ugly side effect called heart-valve disease was disclosed by an article in the *New England Journal of Medicine*. The name Redux entered the weight loss controversy. The fen-phen fiasco may have been swept under a rug, if not for an EKG technician in a small medical clinic in Fargo, ND. After reading the tech's file, the clinic's cardiologists took the data to the Mayo Clinic. What was the outcome? The FDA took it off the market in 1997. Many people had died of internal bleeding. According to current reports, it cost the drug manufacturer, Wyeth, $13 billion to $16 billion in lawsuits. Wyeth is currently attempting to settle all of the claims for the additional cost of $4 billion.

It took decades for scientists to develop treatments that control the dreaded diseases of cholera, diphtheria, polio, and smallpox. We spend billions of dollars in the research and treatment for cancer and heart disease. With billions of dollars going into research and treatments, there's no cure yet for AIDS (40 million deaths and 40 million living with HIV since 1981). Now we are facing the most feared disease of all—Alzheimer's.

While they're trying to discover the treatment or cure for AD, scientists have dropped another "time bomb" on our plate, genetically engineered foods or genetically modified organisms, GMOs. The co-risk factors for AD include the water we drink, the air we breathe, our cookware, our medication, and mineral-depleted soils, to name a few. What new disease will we face after consuming GMO foods for years? Currently the foods we consume or don't consume become AD co-risk factors.

Will GMO foods become a co-risk factor?

Countries such as Austria, Australia, Brazil, China, France, India, Japan, the Philippines, and Egypt are a few of the more than 20 countries that have banned or restricted the import, distribution, sale, utilization, field trials or commercial planting of GMOs. However, the United States does not even require identity or labeling of a GMO ingredient by the US Government and FDA. Actually, more than 75% of our food, animals, and plants in the US have GMOs. The US Department of Agriculture allowed the use of GMOs to increase crop yields, increase product size, decrease insects, etc., with no regard for nutrition. To date, there are twenty US states, numerous counties, and a few cities that ban GE/GMO foods. In 2018 Monsanto went through its first class-action lawsuit where the jury awarded a cancer patient $289 million due to glyphosate (in Roundup), which they produce. Note: Monsanto developed Agent Orange for the federal government. They are a multinational agrochemical and agricultural biotechnology corporation located in St. Louis. The producer of genetically engineered crops (seeds), and pesticides merged with Bayer AG (chemicals and pharmaceuticals) in a $63 billion agreement.

The federal government finally discovered that our financial institutions are too big to control, too big to allow to fail. Can we say this about the giant corporations that control our food supply? Can we trust them? Are their interests centered on greed or the health and well-being of mankind? Are they becoming too big to control?

As for me, I'm not going to worry about it. Our family will continue our periodic checkups by our medical doctors. We will also continue taking supplements to maintain our health and well-being. I call it an investment. We invest in a nice car. We invest in a home. We invest in our children's future, their education. We invest in our future. Is there any reason we should not invest in our health? Without our health, our other investments would become insignificant.

I have known people who came close to dying, but their herbal, mineral, and vitamin supplements saved their lives. That's very unusual, because generally supplements take longer because they build the immune system for the *prevention* of diseases.

During my investigation of AD I found the following contributing risk factors—co-risk factors—mentioned by research scientists, including medical doctors (www.alzinfo.org/research/alzheimers-research-on-causes-and-risk-factors):

- Age
- Zinc
- Bacteria
- Diuretics
- NSAIDs
- Sedatives
- Smoking
- Sleep apnea
- Vaccinations
- High cholesterol
- Cardiac-digoxin
- Solvent absorption
- Years of education
- High blood pressure
- Selenium deficiency
- Vitamin D deficiency
- Heart-bypass surgery
- Aluminum absorption
- Iron balance (low and high)
- Low vitamin B_3
- Aspartame
- Electromagnetic field/impulse power from electrical devices
- Genetic

- Medication (anti-anxiety, antidepressants, antihistamines, anti-spasmodics, anti-psychotics, and more)

Sleep apnea may be new to many readers. However, 30 to 80% of elderly adults suffer from sleep apnea. Many are not aware. It is a sleep disorder with breathing and obstructive sleep apnea, which are associated with amyloid deposition, a biomarker of dementia. They are also associated with Alzheimer's disease (Research presented at the Alzheimer's Association International Conference of 2017 in London). Snoring and sleep apnea are linked to memory loss, as they restrict oxygen to the brain. Those with sleep apnea may face a higher chance of developing AD down the road (Dr. Ricardo Osorio, Assistant Professor of Psychiatry at New York University School of Medicine in New York City). Research into sleep apnea is carried out at medical centers in Amsterdam, Netherlands.

PATIENT PROFILES: PEOPLE I KNEW/ KNOW AND FAMILY MEMBERS

A. Female—author Allen's mother; diagnosed at 74, died at 84. Born in 1909, grew up on the family farm near Newberg, Oregon. Married a logger and lived in a logging camp and logging towns; no indoor plumbing or telephone until she was 36 years old. Hard worker on family farm. Husband died from heart attack at age 55; never remarried. In good health until diagnosed with AD. Co-risk factors: age, aluminum absorption, pernicious anemia (vitamin B_{12} deficiency), brain not challenged. Had two children and one surgery.

B. Male—diagnosed at 67, died from cancer in 2014 at age 80. Worked as a logger, timber feller, excellent health, very nutritional diet consisting of proper amounts of fruits and vegetables, meat was chicken and fish, never more than one beer per day, never smoked, chewed tobacco (had mouth cancer), 10 mg Aricept, various herbal products, very low cholesterol, blood pressure (low end), no electronics, enjoyed TV Westerns, aluminum absorption, played cards well, competitive in timber events, outdoorsman, hunter, worked in large flower and vegetable garden. Co-risk factors: age, aluminum absorption, selenium deficiency, solvents (chain, power saws).

C. Female—diagnosed at 76, died in 2011 at 84. Born in the suburbs of London; family was poor with minimal nutrition before and during World War II; did not drink alcohol or smoke, took numerous pain medications, no problem with high cholesterol or high blood pressure, consumed large amounts of sugar in her tea, fell as a youngster and hit her head on concrete sidewalk (late in life surgery in the US for stomach problems revealed the stomach of a 14-year-old), selenium deficiency (cattle and plant food—refer to the Mad Cow report to Parliament by H. Fullerton, PhD). Co-risk factors: age, brain trauma, selenium deficiency; inflammation (pain medications); secluded lifestyle; limited nutrition in early life.

D. Female—author Allen's wife; diagnosed at 72, died from massive infection at 79 in 2013. Born in 1933; family moved from Minnesota to California, then Oregon; lived in Oregon more than 60 years. In her early life, she endured the harsh winters of International Falls, Minnesota, with temperatures that got down to 30 to 50 degrees below zero; enjoyed large family gatherings and her grandparents' farm; nutritional diet consisted of home-grown produce plus wild game—fish, geese, and venison. Family relocated numerous times before she was 12 years old. Co-risk factors: aluminum absorption, selenium deficiency, periodontitis, high blood pressure, high cholesterol, heart-bypass surgery, sleep apnea, smoking (30-plus years), alcohol (30-plus years), electronic devices.

Note: Her brother died at 76 in 2012. He had a brilliant mind, was a three-sport star athlete in high school; college graduate in business; major cardiovascular health problems. Co-risk factors for AD: age, aluminum absorption, selenium deficiency, high blood pressure, very high cholesterol, heart-bypass surgery, smoking (50-plus years), alcohol (50-plus years). *Yet no indication of AD.*

E. Female—born in Oregon in 1949; lived in farming and logging communities before settling in Portland; active in church on various committees; diagnosed with AD at 60 years old. Co-risk factors: aluminum absorption, selenium deficiency, second-hand smoke.

F. Female—diagnosed at 53. Co-risk factors: alcoholic, aluminum absorption, selenium deficiency, brain not challenged. Currently in AD facility.

G. Female—diagnosed in her late 70s. Co-risk factors: aluminum absorption, selenium deficiency, brain not challenged. Currently in AD facility.

H. Male—Co-author Siler's husband. Born 1936; gifted athlete in three sports in high school; star high school quarterback; junior college scholarship; University of Oregon scholarship; Played in Rose Bowl 1958; high school and college athletic coach; very active social life; golfer, numerous hobbies including boating, fishing, woodworking. Co-risk factors: age, aluminum absorption, brain trauma (high school QB, college receiver), selenium deficiency.

I. Male—diagnosed with dementia at age 90, died at 91; PhD, Psychiatry, brain researcher, UCLA, Stanford. Co-risk factors: age, aluminum absorption, selenium deficiency.

J. Male—born 1939, died in 2018 at 79; diagnosed in 2016. Grew up in the Pacific Northwest, US Navy tour of duty; Portland State University, BA; Oregon State University. MA; educator, pilot, great physical condition as runner. Co-risk factors: age, aluminum absorption, selenium deficiency.

K. Female—diagnosed at 87, died at 94; retired teacher; non-smoker; non-drinker. Co-risk factors: age, aluminum absorption, selenium deficiency.

L. Male—diagnosed at 85, died at 92; farmer; organic food, non-smoker, non-drinker. Co-risk factors: age, aluminum absorption, selenium deficiency.

M. Male (son of the male above)—diagnosed at 75, died at 82; consumed processed foods; smoked cigarettes; drank alcohol. Co-risk factors: age, aluminum absorption, selenium deficiency, diet, smoking, alcohol.

As reported in the *Archives of General Psychiatry*, having a purpose in life is associated with a decreased risk of developing Alzheimer's disease, mild cognitive impairment, and a slower rate of cognitive decline. ("A Purposeful Life Decreases the Risk of Alzheimer's" by Aron S. Buchman, *Archives of General Psychiatry*, March 12, 2010)

Heart problems such as heart-bypass surgery, high blood pressure, high cholesterol, and vascular disorders are co-risk factors in developing Alzheimer's disease. The February 11, 2018, edition of *The Oregonian* included Life's Simple 7—if not corrected, these health issues can also cause a heart attack.

The following information on blood pressure, provided by Regence, was also included in *The Oregonian* story. The American College of Cardiology and the American Heart Association have new guidelines that lower the threshold for a high blood pressure diagnosis. The old threshold was 140/90. The new threshold is 130/80.

QUESTIONNAIRE
Co-Risk Factors Concentration (none/low/moderate/high)

- *Age seventy at diagnosis
- *Aluminum absorption
- Aspartame
- *Blood pressure
- *Brain trauma
- *Cardiac-digoxin
- Cholesterol

- Dioxin
- Diuretics
- *Drugs, NSAID, etc.
- Advil
- Aleve
- Aspirin
- Bayer

---

* Most common co-risk

- Celebrex
- Ibuprofen
- Indocin
- Motrin
- Naproxen
- Nuprin
- Opiates—codeine, et al.
- Toradol
- Vaprosyn
- Electronic devises
- *Fluoride absorption
- Fumigants
- Genetics
- *Heart-bypass surgery
- Homocysteine
- *Infections—UTI, etc.
- *Menopause-early
- Inflammation
- Depression
- *Gum disease– periodontitis
- Low carb diet
- *Social stress
- PTSD
- *Sleep apnea—poor sleep quality
- *IQ
- Medications
- Mineral balance
- Iron
- *Selenium—deficient
- Smoking
- *Solvents
- Adhesives
- Alcohols
- Benzene
- Ketones
- Paints
- Phenols
- Toluene
- Xylene
- Statin drugs
- Tap water (lead)
- Vitamin deficiency
- *Vitamin B complex
- *Vitamin B_{12}
- Vitamin D

---

* Most common co-risk

CHAPTER 10

SUGGESTED NUTRITION

YOUR TOTAL CO-RISK FACTORS
(top co-risk factors—an unscientific opinion)

In the United States we have two groups of health professionals. One group embraces the prevention of illness—that of getting well and staying well. The other group encourages treatments to get well *after* being stricken with an illness. They actually depend on you and me to get sick and request their services. They are the medical professionals who embrace the pharmaceutical industry and their synthetic drugs.

Example: The dilemma of the flu shot. To have or not to have? Myself...I have built up my immune system over the years by proper nutrition, exercise, periodic check-ups from my MD, plus supplements (herbal formulations, minerals, vitamins), as well as consuming my share of processed snack food. I follow my MD's advice and receive the required flu plus any other shot. It's good insurance for wellness. When I travel overseas I carry a travel kit with a number of supplements (which includes my number one herb pau d'arco—a super-antibiotic). My first time staying in an

American hotel in China (Holiday Inn) was one to remember. Half of the hotel guests came down with a strain of the Hong Kong flu. I felt a bit woozy for only a day, thanks to my kit plus the flu shot I received before I left home. I have faith in the AMA, FDA and Big Pharma to guide me. It would be very stupid of me to waste my life ingesting products that harm me—excess alcohol, junk food, harmful (street) drugs, while wasting away as a couch potato. When I'm a hopeless mental and physical mess, it's too late to call upon the Big Three to bail me out! It's up to me to treat my body with respect. It's the only body I have. In 2016, 13% of the US population encountered the flu. That's not bad considering we had 76 million international visitors who are not screened for an infectious disease. An infection advances AD a year or more. (Stats are from Federal government research.)

An article in the September 8, 2011, issue of *The Oregonian* brought out a cozy deal Big Pharma has with our nation's medical doctors. ("Oregon Doctors Get Millions in Drug Pay" by Nick Budnick, *The Oregonian*, September 8, 2011; "Drugmakers Tossed $6.5 Billion Doctors' Way" *The Washington Post*, reported in *The Oregonian*, July 6, 2016) They retain them as "consultants." The doctors travel on behalf of a pharmaceutical firm to speak and conduct seminars promoting the firm's products. They are akin to shills. Note the TV ads displaying this unusual marketing tool ... "Ask your doctor if you should be using Xamasik." What's this? They are asking us to self-diagnose? I've been told that is a no-no. They may serve on the firm's advisory board. Since 2009, Lilly has paid one Oregon doctor over $135,000. GlaxoSmithKline paid another Oregon doctor over $226,000. Pfizer was also listed as a pharmaceutical company paying Oregon doctors to peddle their products. The total outlay for pharmaceutical "lobbyists" was nearly $800 million between 2009 and 2018.

I wonder if that includes the monies that are "invested" in medical students for tuition and expenses. There are those in the federal government who say this practice affects the cost of health care. Look who's calling the kettle black. Do they believe Washington lobbyists keep our government on an ethical track? It's their ethics, not the taxpayer's. What about the politicians and generals who retire and take lucrative positions with the Pentagon, a federal agency, or a defense contractor? Is that not a strategy to influence contracts and regulations?

JAMA (*Journal of the American Medical Association*) published a statement in their January 3, 1959, issue penned by their Council on Foods and Nutrition. The subject? The use of vitamin preparations as dietary supplements and as therapeutic agents. The media jumped on the chance to run interference for the AMA. They penned headlines such as, "Vitamins and Food Supplements Declared by AMA Not Necessary and Perhaps Harmful."

Their Council on Foods and Nutrition claims an adequate diet that meets the government Recommended Dietary Allowance (RDA) will maintain one's health. Most nutritional professionals outside of government and the AMA consider the government RDAs as that amount sufficient for a living person with a pulse to "fog a mirror."

A study from the 1970s revealed that a startling number of Americans were chronically ill—more than 90 million. No doubt a current study would reveal that number to exceed 150 million—around 50% of our population. It is impossible for the average American to maintain good health without taking supplements. Any person who can listen, observe, and read realizes the nutritional deficiencies we all face. For example, if our school lunches are so great, why do our youngsters have the highest obesity rates in the world? Why do many housewives live on desserts, starches, coffee, and fats? Why do we have vending machines dispensing junk food in our schools?

The US government stresses adherence to established guidelines for food choices to balance calories with physical activity.

Maintaining one's weight is one effort to lower the incidence of chronic diseases. Nutrition is considered the main factor in preventing chronic diseases. Once one has been afflicted by a disease, nutrition is part of the therapy to regain one's health. That said, our government has failed its citizens miserably. Statistics reveal that we have the most obese citizens of any nation in the world. When it comes to nutrition, I doubt if 50% of our high school students could pass a test on the function of vitamins. I doubt if 50% know *what* food products supply *which* vitamins. And we worry about our students' lack of knowledge in mathematics and science. They lack the basic know-how to plan well-balanced meals for proper nutrition. Their menu choices in a restaurant ignore proper nutrition.

I have made a few presentations on cardiovascular diseases and their prevention at senior citizen meetings and retirement home luncheons. A few of the people with heart problems asked me to check off on the facility calendar which meals were best for their type of diet. I doubt if 10% of the meals served at their facility would be rated acceptable by a dietitian. The meals were loaded with calories in the form of pasta, cheese, mashed potatoes and gravy, pizza, etc. In one month of lunches, they served a chef salad only one day. Other salad options were not listed.

We lunched at our favorite seafood restaurant at least twice a week. My favorites are a crab or shrimp Louie or a Caesar salad with a bowl of clam chowder or fisherman's stew, with the salads being the half portion. My wife's favorite was the pear, pecan, blue cheese chunks with grilled chicken strips, salad—a half portion. We found this adequate and filling, especially with the Italian bread they served. However, many people who weigh at least 250 pounds order the full salad, bowl of chowder, the bread, a beer or a couple glasses of wine, plus a dessert. And they wonder why they can't lose weight?

If you have no reference to the list of thirty-four nutrients and what their deficiency could cause, try to obtain the list (pages 31–38) from Dr. Ladd McNamara's *Medical Resource Manual, Fourth Edition*—The Importance of Nutrition & The Consequences of Deficiencies.

The FDA has revised the labels of food products to provide more detailed information on nutrition ("FDA Hopes to Fight Obesity by Revising Nutrition Labels" by Shaya Tayefe Mohajer, The Associated Press, asreported in *The Oregonian*, September 4, 2011).

Here's the current typical label on a package of turkey smoked sausage: They list the ingredients, dates on when to use or freeze once opened, that it's fully cooked, keep refrigerated, heat and serve. If the buyer can read, it's self-explanatory.

Does the buyer read the label?
Nutrition facts on the label: serving size, 2 oz.; calories, 90; fat calories, 45; total fat, 5g (sat. fat 1.5g, trans fat, 0g); cholesterol, 30mg; sodium, 500mg (21%); total carbs, 3g; fiber less than 1g; sugars, 1g; protein, 9g; calcium, 2%; iron 4%.

Does the buyer read this info?
The FDA proposes changes on the label that would include "more accurate serving sizes, a greater emphasis on calories, and a diminished role in the daily percent values for substances like fat, sodium, and carbohydrates."

More current labels:
Popular brand of green beans—Nutrition facts: serving size, ½ cup; calories, 25; total fat, 0g; saturated fat, 0g; trans. fat, 0g; cholesterol, 0g; sodium, 270mg (11%); carbs, 5g; dietary fiber, 1g; sugars, 1g, protein, 0g; vitamin A, 4%, Iron, 2%.

Popular brand of black beans (50% less sodium)—Nutrition facts: serving size, ½ cup; calories, 120; total fat, 0.5g; saturated fat, 0g; trans. fat, 0g; cholesterol, 0mg; sodium, 180mg (8%); carbs, 22g; dietary fiber, 5g (20%); sugars, 1g; calcium, 6%; iron, 10%.

Popular brand of enchilada sauce—Nutrition facts: serving size, ¼ cup; calories, 20; total fat, 0g; cholesterol, 0g; sodium, 330mg (14%); carbs, 4g; dietary fiber, 0g; sugars, 1g; protein, 1g; vitamin A, 4%; vitamin C, 70%; iron, 2%.

I wonder if anybody at the FDA ever had to shop for groceries on a budget. Maybe they shop for the top brand regardless of sodium content, cholesterol, carbs, fat, and sugar. I do all the shopping in our family at two major supermarkets when they feature their sales, Thursday through Saturday. Have you noticed when shopping for chili that there are at least a dozen and a half varieties? Are you going to read every label? Of course not. If every shopper read each label in selecting, they would spend at least two hours in the market, causing a severe shopper jam. As with chili, do you want no beans, beef, chicken, turkey, or vegan chili? The sodium will range from 840 to 1400 mg for a cup—half the can. The contents vary from 14.5 ounces to 15.5 ounces, though they appear to be the same size. So which one is the best buy and best nutrition for your family? Personally, I make my own chili (option A: If I'm in a hurry, I mix a 15.5 oz. can of S&W black chili beans (480 mg sodium) and a 15 oz. can of WinCo chili beans (540 mg sodium)—half the cost and half the sodium (510 mg). Option B: I mix a 15 oz. can of Hormel chili no beans (990 mg sodium, 250 calories) and a 15.5 oz. can of S&W chili beans (190 mg sodium, 130 calories) for an average 590 mg sodium and half the calories). The store-bought chili has too much sodium for my taste. Sodium is also a preservative. I read the stamped can that indicates items processed in 2008 are best used by 2014—that's a six-year shelf-life. Most of the canned foods that I have used contained too much salt. Their excess salt is added for a longer shelf-life. A few food companies go so far as to note: Add salt for taste.

The FDA is assuming the grocery shopper is capable of making good decisions on nutrition. With a 49% rate of low literacy and a 14% rate of illiteracy among American adults, according to US government statistics, a large percentage of the American grocery shoppers cannot make good decisions on nutrition. Unfortunately, these are probably the people who have the problem of being overweight. While I'm shopping at the two large supermarkets, I noticed that many of the shoppers are overweight. Occasionally, I shop at a small market that is more like a deli, no meat or produce other than prepackaged. I shop there because they feature items not stocked at the large markets; however, the prices can be higher, though not always. The majority of the shoppers appear young with lean bodies. They look as if they just dropped in from a 20-mile bike ride or an hour in the gym. In my opinion, a revised food label may be the wrong place to correct an overweight problem among our people. It should begin in the classrooms and cafeterias of our schools.

I consider myself in good health for my age. However, I owe most of it to the start my body received as a youngster. I was not one to pick up every germ that slithered down the pike such as colds and flu. My first major disease was infantile paralysis (now known as polio) at the age of 18 months, a mild case. Of course, I had all the childhood diseases—chicken pox, measles, and mumps. From the time I began my career with a Fortune 500 firm until retirement, I cannot remember a day that I stayed home due to illness—other than a mild heart attack at age 37 due to my high-stress job, but there was no damage.

As a youngster, I preferred raw vegetables. When Mom prepared dinner, which would include cooked carrots, cauliflower, turnips, or other vegetables, she set my portion aside, and I ate it raw. My typical snack was raw carrots, celery, turnips, and tomatoes. Potato chips, pie, cake, cookies, and candy were a treat. Until I was 18 years old, my parents had a small farm where we raised our own chickens (for eggs and meat), a cow (for milk and cream), and a pig (for meat, ham smoked by Dad). Our fruit was all natural, organic from the local small farms: gooseberries, raspberries, strawberries, blackberries, peaches, and plums. (Mom made sure our fridge/pantry was stocked with apples, bananas, and oranges out of season.) It was a trend in high school to be cool and eat pomegranates at a nickel a pop. Little did we know it is one of the best antioxidants. We were also blessed with local filberts (hazelnuts are the wild variety), and walnuts. Add to this nature's bounty from the streams and rivers: wild trout and salmon. Razor clams from the beach and venison from a deer hunt made for extremely nutritional food compared to what the majority of Americans youngsters consume today. I enjoyed vegetables from our own garden until I left home at 18 and married. Throughout my adult life, our family has enjoyed good nutritional food along with the occasional fast-food from Burger King, KFC, and Chinese takeout. However, since the 1990s our family has been on a regimen of herbal, mineral, and vitamin formulation supplements.

GMO foods—Before I proceed with the topic of this chapter on nutrition, I will bring you up to date on GMO (genetically modified organisms) foods. According to the US Department of Agriculture, GMO foods were primarily approved for insect and herbicide resistance. Additional benefits could include improved yield, appearance and size, reduced maturing time, increased shelf life, stress tolerance, altered taste and texture. After 30 years, the USDA admits they concentrated too much on insect and herbicide resistance. Currently, the most common GMO foods include alfalfa, canola, corn, and soybeans. Since 2006, 53% of food in US contains GMOs, including 93% of soybeans and 70% of corn. Animals are fed genetically modified high fructose corn syrup. Bacon, burgers, cheese, dairy, ice cream, meat: all contain GMOs. The worst foods with GMOs are corn, soy, canola (canola oil advances Alzheimer's), sugar, aspartame (a known carcinogen, a co-risk factor in Alzheimer's), yellow crookneck squash and zucchini, alfalfa, sugar beets (half of US sugar production, 95% of

US market), and milk. Many cows in the US are given genetically engineered recombinant bovine growth hormone (rBGH), which is banned in Australia, Canada, the EU, Japan, and New Zealand. The situation has been improving, though, and a US Department of Agriculture survey conducted in 2007 found that less than 1 in 5 cows (17%) were being injected with rBGH. Monsanto produces Roundup, which contains glyphosate, a toxic herbicide. Monsanto is in the discussion phase with the USDA to reintroduce 2,4-D, a component of Agent Orange.

Note: The federal government is paying hundreds of millions of dollars to the Vietnamese government for the health damage Agent Orange caused to the environment (soils) and people of Vietnam. Additionally, 200,000 Vietnam US veterans suffer health problems related to Agent Orange. And Monsanto wants to reintroduce it? Are they insane? The USDA would be insane to approve it.

A non-GMO ear of corn will supply 6% RDA for vitamin C, 10% RDA for fiber, and 3 grams of protein. One cup will supply 15% RDA for folic acid, and 12% RDA for vitamin B_3.

I could find no data on the nutritional value of GMO corn. However, in 2009, Dr. Chuxia Deng, editor, *International Journal of Biological Science* (a position with the National Institutes of Health), reported the side effects of GMO corn on laboratory rats. Their adrenal glands, heart, kidney, liver, and spleen all encountered severe problems.

In December 2012, the FDA approved the GMO Atlantic salmon that will reach market weight in 18 months rather than 36. The salmon was developed by AquaBounty in Massachusetts. A recent article from Norway put my mind at ease. They have perfected a fish farm process that could feed the world with salmon, without GMOs. If you favor Atlantic salmon check it out. Myself, I was raised on Chinook (Pacific, King, Tyee) salmon. Plus, I have caught my share of salmon—Chinook and Coho off the coast of Oregon and Washington, and King salmon in the Kenai River in Alaska.

GMO apples have been under review by USDA since 2010. Okanagan Specialty Fruits, Inc. of British Columbia developed apples that will not turn brown for an entire two weeks, after slicing. McDonald's and Gerber's have not rejected their Arctic apples. Cherries, peaches, and pears are next in line for GMO technology.

Now some more disturbing news about GMO foods. "World's Number 1 Herbicide Discovered in US Mothers' Breast Milk" (Sustainable Pulse, April 6, 2014). Studies show a build-up of glyphosate herbicide in mothers' bodies. Urine testing shows glyphosate levels over ten times higher than in Europe. Monsanto has a warning in the 21-page booklet for their Roundup: *Dispose of wastes in an approved landfill.* However, when used to kill weeds, etc., it seeps into the ground. Rains and sprinkling flush it into city storm drains and eventually into streams, rivers, fish habitat, and our municipal water supply. Glyphosate is found in our water systems. As of this writing, Monsanto is involved in class action lawsuits over glyphosate causing cancers.

Dr. Arpad Pusztai (b. 1930) is a Hungarian-born biochemist and nutritionist. He earned a PhD in chemistry from Eotvos Lorand University in Budapest, and a PhD in biochemistry from the University of London. He worked for 36 years with Scotland's Rowett Research Institute, and also for the Lister Institute of Preventive Medicine in London. He is a Fellow of Royal Society of Edinburgh. After the 1999 publication in *The Lancet* of a controversial research paper on mineral and vitamin loss in GMO foods that argued GMO potatoes had a negative effect on rats' stomachs and immune systems, Dr. Pusztai lost his position at Rowett. In 2005, he received the Whistleblower Award from the International Association of Lawyers Against Nuclear Arms and the Federation of German Scientists. In 2009, Dr. Pusztai and his wife, professor Bardocz Zsuzsa, were awarded the Stuttgart Peace Prize.

"The continued cultivation of GM crops increases the use of toxic pesticides, herbicides, and fertilizers, which leach into soil as well as circulates in the air. Studies show that herbicide use increased by 527 million pounds between 1996 and 2011, other studies project that number to increase thirty-fold between 2011 and 2019. While scientists may not fully understand the long-term health impact from consuming GM food, we do know that many of these chemicals do several things. They corrupt and deteriorate the human microbiome, leading to heavy growth of unhealthy bacteria and the displacement of healthy bacteria, potentially linked to increasing rates of ADHD [glyphosate-Roundup], and potentially linked to rising rates of neurological disorders [chlorpyrifos]. GMOs endure because their seeds can't be removed from the environment and their spreading in the environment can't be fully controlled" ("As Mother Nature Intended" by Lisa Schofield, *Nutrition Industry Executive*, June 2017).

Note: Chlorpyrifos was introduced in 1965 by Dow Chemical; Glyphosate was introduced in 1974 by Monsanto.

The majority of medical doctors in America are drug-oriented. They are beholden to the AMA, Big Pharma, and FDA, which preach that supplements (herbs, minerals, vitamins) are not necessary. Some even go so far as to say, they are "snake oil," they will kill you, or are a waste of money. Nutrition alone is ideal, if you can be sure of the minerals and vitamins your food contains.

Why is Big Pharma nervous, and why have the AMA, Big Pharma, and FDA been bad-mouthing the supplement industry in the past few years? For openers, the patents on a number of their "billion dollar pills" have expired. Revenues of $2 to $6 billion a year per pill have gone bye-bye. Their loss of total revenue since 2012 is nearly $28 billion. Adding to their dilemma is the fact that more seniors and baby boomers are leaning more to supplements to maintain their health and well-being.

The Ohio Agricultural Experiment Station in Wooster, Ohio,

published a research paper in 1957 titled, "Nutritional Status of 9-, 10-, and 11-year-old Public School Children in Iowa, Kansas, and Ohio." The children had their blood tested for hemoglobin, vitamin C, vitamin A, and carotene. They were found to be deficient by 36 to 56%. They were not children from poor families. They were not children from a Third World nation. They were American children from the food basket of America. Our farmland soils are deficient of essential minerals and vitamins.

An internationally recognized pediatrician from Oregon took his family on a vacation to Europe in the early 1990s. Being an advocate of nutritional supplements, the MD collected soil samples from the farmlands they visited in France, Germany, and Italy. Back in Oregon, he collected soil samples from our Willamette Valley farmlands and had all of the samples tested at Oregon State University laboratories. Confirming his assumption, the soils from the Willamette Valley were revealed to be the most deficient in nutrients (minerals and vitamins).

Perhaps one of the best articles on soil depletion is by T.J. Clark of Australia. Their study reveals that farmlands of America are depleted by a range of 60 to 100%. Research by the University of Texas at Austin's Department of Chemistry and Biochemistry was published in the *Journal of the American College of Nutrition,* December 2004. They studied data from the US Department of Agriculture from 1950 and 1999 for 43 various vegetables and fruit, revealing declines in the amounts of protein, calcium, iron, phosphorus, riboflavin, and vitamin C over the past half century. They contribute this action to the agricultural practice designed to improve traits like size, growth rate, and pest resistance instead of nutrition. As one scientist so aptly phrased it: "One would have to eat eight oranges today to derive the same amount of Vitamin C as grandma got from one."

While fertile land in America has been "farmed to death," nutrients that are taken from the soil in crops *are not being replaced.* Chemical fertilizers contain certain minerals, but soils must contain many more, such as trace minerals that are lacking in crops from these soils. *Fertilizers are the problem, not the solution.* According to Gary Price Todd, MD, the human body requires at least 60 minerals, 12 essential amino acids, 16 vitamins, and 3 essential fatty acids for optimal health. A plant cannot manufacture copper, molybdenum, or zinc. It can only take it from the soil in which it grows. So where are future generations of Americans going to get these trace minerals under our current methods of farming? There are only two sources—organically grown food from enriched soils and nutritional supplements.

Dr. Linus Pauling, founder of the Linus Pauling Institute at Oregon State University, stated that all ailments, diseases, and sicknesses *are the result of mineral deficiency.*

Take note of the information printed on the packaging of the food products on the shelves of our supermarkets. They contain added minerals and vitamins, no doubt because of the research conducted by the Ohio group in 1957. The most common additives are vitamin A and C, plus calcium and iron. On the more expensive breakfast cereals you will find at least 14, as well as the top brand pasta which contains 14 mineral and vitamin additives.

Now, check out the dog food you buy for Max or Mindy—at least 20 to 40 supplements are added. Hey, they can't trot to their local pet health food shop and pick up a bottle of alfalfa, He-Shou-Wu, and Siberian ginseng.

Christa Orecchio, Clinical and Holistic Nutritionist, has a website called *The Whole Journey* that may be helpful. Her work also led me to Dr. Peter D'Adamo, who has authored a good reference book called *The Blood Type Diet.* Here are suggested brief guidelines to consider:

Type A: People with this blood type are better at extracting protein from vegetarian sources. They should consume less red meat, dairy, wheat, and kidney beans. They should include foods high in vitamins C and E, folic acid, and immune boosters that include fruits, vegetables, miso, tempeh, whole grains, legumes, and seafood. Those who are vegan/vegetarian should supplement their diet with vitamin B_{12}.

Type AB: This is the rarest of all blood types. Their mixed diet should include meat (not red meat), seafood, beans, legumes, high-quality dairy, vegetables, and fruit. People with this blood type do not process corn, kidney beans, or red meat very well.

Type B: Those with this blood type do best by avoiding corn, peanuts, wheat, and seeds. Eggs, greens, and most animal meats are great to include in their diet.

Type O: People with this blood type do better without corn, wheat, or pasteurized dairy in their diet. They also react poorly to kidney beans and Brussels sprouts. Their best foods are high-quality grass-fed beef, kelp, seafood, spinach, broccoli, and kale.

Countless articles and books listing the nutrition for optimal health include the following foods:

Fish—Wild salmon (has less dioxin than farm-raised salmon), halibut, albacore tuna, and lake trout. Shrimp and lobster were considered foods to avoid due to cholesterol. Not true. Shrimp is a good source for protein, vitamin B_3, D, and zinc. Lobster is a good source for protein, vitamins B and F, phosphorus, magnesium, and zinc.

Meats—Chicken, lamb, pork, veal, beef (in moderation).

Fruits—Organic apples, blackberries, blueberries, cherries, pears, and persimmons.

Vegetables—Broccoli, brown rice, butternut squash, kale, spinach, sweet potato, grape tomatoes.

Nuts—almonds, filberts/hazelnuts, peanuts (actually a legume), and walnuts.

Crisp breads—Ry Krisp, Ryvita, Wasa. They are loaded with fiber, and often fat-free.

Beverages—Blueberry, Concord grape, and pomegranate juice,

milk (almond, coconut, skim), and green tea. Green tea has been found to have health benefits. Researchers at the University of Basel (Switzerland) are revealing the first evidence that green tea extract enhances the cognitive functions, in particular the working memory ("Green Tea Boosts the Brain, Nutrition" *Industry Executive*, May 2014). Our salt intake must be closely monitored. Try to limit your daily sodium intake to 1,500 mg for people over 50 (note that most frozen dinners from the markets exceed this amount in one serving), African Americans of any age, and people who have high blood pressure, diabetes, or chronic kidney disease. Sugar should be avoided. Foods have enough sugar.

When buying canned fruit, buy fruit canned in water or very light syrup.

Cheese is not good for optimum brain health. Hard cheese is okay in small quantities. For a "buttery spread" use butter or Smart Balance, which contains beta-carotene, lecithin, folic acid, omega-3 (ALA, EPA/DHA) and vitamins A, B_6, B_{12}, and D. All of my cooking is with grape seed oil, olive oil (extra virgin), or coconut oil (tolerates more heat). Less than 10% of your calories should come from saturated fatty acids. Our daily limit of cholesterol is 300 mg, which could be exceeded by only 3.5 ounces of beef kidney. In alcohol consumption, the daily limit for men is two drinks, for women, one, as established by numerous US government agencies. This amount is debated by British, French, and Swedish medical researchers.

Vitamin D—Thinking, learning, and memory decline in older adults with low vitamin D. A six-year study of 900 adults, age 65 and older, revealed a severe deficiency in 60% of those having cognitive decline. (Llewellyn DJ et al. Vitamin D and risk of cognitive decline in elderly persons. *Arch Intern Med* 2010 Jul 12: 170(13):1135-41.) Estimates in Europe and the US place 40 to 100% of older adults with vitamin D deficiency. They link this to fractures, chronic disease, and death. Other studies confirm that up to half of the US population may be deficient. A combination of nutrition, exposure to sunlight and supplements will provide normal levels of vitamin D, 50ng/ml. A blood test will reveal your Vitamin D level. Vitamin D is found in oily fish (salmon, mackerel, sardines); cod liver oil; cereals (fortified); skim milk (fortified); and eggs. About fifteen minutes of sunlight absorbed through the scalp and other areas seems to be sufficient. A form of vitamin D_3 with curcumin (the main ingredient in turmeric) may stimulate the body's immune system to clear amyloid beta from the brain. The vitamin D supplement should include magnesium, zinc, boron, genistein, vitamin A, and vitamin $_{K2}$.

Vitamin E—Researchers at the Minneapolis Veterans Administration Health Care System say vitamin E might slow down the progression of mild to moderate AD. A study of 600 older veterans revealed a decrease in the rate of progression (M. Marchione, Associated Press, 2014). Natural d-alpha tocopherol and d-gamma tocopherol mix have the most benefit. A deficiency may be a co-risk factor in Alzheimer's, the progression of AD, asthma, cancer, diabetes, heart disease, low immune system, etc. To best absorb vitamin E, take it with food.

Selenium—Before 1957, selenium was considered toxic and thought to be carcinogenic. Current research has found it to be anti-carcinogenic. In the late 1960s, surveys found soils of the Pacific Northwest, upper Midwest, Northeast and along the Atlantic coast do not contain enough selenium to supply adequate plant growth for feeding animals. (LPI, Selenium and Cancer: *New Views*, LPI Newsletter, Fall/Winter, 1997). Selenium is an antioxidant trace mineral found in plants, animals, and seafood with specific fish having the highest content. There are scientists who claim that fish in our diet should be limited to one serving a week due to mercury in fish. However, other scientists claim the selenium in fish eliminates the effects of mercury. There have been research studies around the globe that reveal low selenium in our diet increases the risk of major health problems, including AIDS, Alzheimer's, cancers, and heart disease. Selenium builds the immune system. The Food and Drug Administration disputes most of the health claims on selenium. The FDA states: "Scientific evidence is convincing, but not yet conclusive." I wonder if they (AMA, Big Pharma and FDA) have a different meaning for the word conclusive when applied to a new drug. Apparently they do, or why would we have over 200,000 deaths a year from adverse drug reactions? The typical amount of selenium taken as a supplement is 50 to 200 mcg. Never exceed a maximum of 400 mcg without monitoring by a health/medical professional.

Calorie restriction is a new trend that could promise a longer, more healthy life. ("Calorie Restriction a Key to Longer Life?" *Vita Journal*, May 2011) The typical American diet may range from 2,000 to 3,000 calories per day. On a severely restricted diet, they suggest 1,800 calories for men and 1,500–1,700 for women. More research is pointing toward calorie restriction as a key to longevity. A 20-year study of laboratory testing (non-humans) revealed reduced risks of cancerous tumors and cardiovascular disease in calorie-restricted diets. To cut calories from your diet: eat less; avoid large portions; enjoy your food, eat slowly; choose low- or, no-fat diary; cut down or eliminate snack foods, fatty meats, and pastries, and consume fresh vegetables and fruit to your heart's content. Complete prevention of diabetes was revealed after calorie reduction. Restricted diets seemed to preserve the areas of the brain involved in motor control, working memory, and problem solving.

"A low fructose diet was recently shown to reduce both blood pressure and inflammation in those with chronic kidney disease, and should be considered an option for anyone with elevated blood pressure." (www.ncbi.nlm.nih.gov)

Score one for those of us who put our faith and judgment in nutrition as the path to greater health and well-being. The founder of Bob's Red Mill Natural Foods near Portland and his wife Charlee pledged $25 million to the Oregon Health & Science University. Their gift has established the Bob and Charlee Moore Institute for Nutrition and Wellness. Also in 2018, the Moores pledged $5 million to Oregon State University to establish a new research and outreach center focusing on nutrition and disease prevention in the College of Health and Human Sciences.

Oregon State University is the home of the Linus Pauling Institute, co-founded in 1973 as the Institute of Orthomolecular Medicine by Linus Pauling (BS, OAC, now OSU; PhD, chemistry, California Institute of Technology) He worked at Cal Tech for 38 years. He is the only individual ever to win two unshared Nobel Prizes. Researchers at LPI investigate what role vitamins, micronutrients, and other dietary constituents, as well as oxidative and nitrative stress and antioxidants play in human aging and chronic diseases—especially heart disease, cancer, and neurodegenerative diseases. Their research can be reviewed at http://lpi.oregonstate.edu. LPI's program is principally supported by gifts from individuals, private corporations, and foundations, grants from federal and private agencies, and from Oregon State University.

From 2000 to 2013, a number of scientists from the Linus Pauling Institute conducted nutritional studies on schoolchildren ages 4 to 13 in a highly educated college city in Oregon. The youngsters were found to have insufficient blood vitamin D, and a diet with insufficient fiber, essential fatty acids, potassium, and vitamin E. They also had excessive saturated fatty acids and sodium. (LPI—Healthy Youth Program, August 2014)

Diet products containing the chemical sweetener aspartame (NutraSweet and Equal) can have multiple neurotoxic, metabolic, allergenic, fetal, and carcinogenic effects. Despite two decades spent analyzing the role of aspartame as a co-risk factor for Alzheimer's, "aspartame disease" has been a largely ignored disorder. The FDA, AMA and many public health/regulatory organizations have ignored the findings. As far back as 1988, seven years after the initial release of aspartame, 80% of the consumer complaints to the FDA concerned aspartame. By April 1995, it had received 7,232 complaints. In many of these complaints, aspartame has been implicated as initiating or aggravating Alzheimer's. Studies indicate aspartame is used by more than 65% of the population. Its original purpose was to treat peptic ulcers. (Google "Aspartame Disease: An FDA-Approved Epidemic" by H. J. Roberts, M.D., F.A.C.P., F.C.C.P., August 12, 2006)

A pair of new studies has been added to the body of evidence supporting a so-called "Mediterranean diet." In one study such a diet was linked to a lower risk of AD. The other study found that the diet could lower the risk of peripheral vascular disease (PVD), a blockage of the veins. The four-year study of 2,258 elderly New Yorkers was conducted by researchers from Columbia University Medical Center, who developed a "Mediterranean diet" index. (As reported in the *Annals of Neurology* online edition, April 18, 2006. Results from the PVD study are included in the article on the InCHIANTI study, *Atherosclerosis*, May 2006, pp 200-206. "Studies: Med diet could protect against Alzheimer's; Vein disorders" *Vitamin Retailer*, June 6, 2006)

When it comes to food we ingest into our body, we should use good judgment. *U.S. News & World Report* ranked the MIND diet the easiest to follow and best diet overall in 2016. (Fend off Alzheimer's and dementia with food, says Liz Applegate, a nutritionist at the University of California-Davis. She stresses the MIND diet—leafy greens, vegetables, nuts, berries, limited red meat, butter, cheese, sweets, and fried foods.) MIND stands for Mediterranean-DASH Intervention for Neurodegenerative Delay. It was developed by Chicago's Rush University Medical Center researchers in 2015. (*Today's Geriatric Medicine*, Nov/Dec 2017)

CHAPTER 11

SUPPLEMENTS—HERBS, MINERALS, VITAMINS

HISTORY OF HERBS—MEDICINAL PLANTS

"I have given you every herb that yields seed which is on the face of all the earth, and every tree whose fruit yields seed; to you it shall be for food."

—Genesis 1:29 NKJV

India: Ayurveda is incorporated into most texts of the Verda, the ancient scriptures upon which Hindu culture and religion are based. It is thought to have existed since 10,000 bc. In the Rigveda over 1,000 medicinal plants are listed. The Indian system, like the Chinese system, works to *maintain health and prevent disease.*

China: Records indicate herbal use back to 5000 bc. Fu Hsi, circa 2852 bc, formulated the theory of yin and yang. Shen Nung, the divine farmer, circa 2697 bc, is considered the father of both agriculture and of herbal medicine. Huang Nei, who lived between 2697 bc and 2595 bc, is thought to be the author of the

Nei Ching, which is still used in China as a medical text. Common Chinese herbs today include aconite, dong quai, He-Shou-Wu, ma huang, pan pien lien, poppy, and rhubarb.

Egypt: Seven hundred herbal remedies dating back to 1500 bc. Medicines of plant origin include celandine, garlic, juniper, lily, linseed, lotus, and thyme.

Greece: Hippocrates, the father of medical literature, had a greater influence than anyone on the direction in which healing and the use of herbs developed in Europe more than 2,500 years ago. Hippocrates' pharmacopoeia included anise, burdock, cinnamon, clove, holy basil, mint, peony, rosemary, thistle, and violet.

Arabia: Herbal shops opened in Baghdad by the early ninth century. Folk remedies and herbal wisdom became a threat to medical academies. By keeping all herbals and pharmacopoeia in Latin, the practice of medicine was controlled by college-trained physicians.

Herbs and plants noted in the Bible (current use):

- Aloe—Used to treat burns, heal rashes, moisturize skin, lower blood sugar, constipation, and decrease liver damage caused by alcohol.
- Anise—Reduces fever/high temperatures and is helpful for COPD.
- Balm or balsam—Herbal salves and oils.
- Bitter herbs—A collective term for horehound, tansy, horseradish, endive, parsley, and coriander seeds. Current herb use: gentian and wormwood—to relieve digestive problems, as well as assisting with blood circulation in the abdominal organs.
- Cassia—Has aromatic properties similar to cinnamon. It is used in natural hair care, coloring, and conditioning.
- Cinnamon—Once considered more precious than gold; collected for anointing oil and perfume. It helps lower

blood glucose levels, is a treatment for yeast infections, an anti-fungal, and calms an upset stomach by relieving gas.

- Cumin—"A cure for everything"—Seeds used to flavor food. It contains a substance useful in fighting diabetes. – Studies have found that black cumin contains an anti-cancer phytochemical; considered a future drug in cancer treatment. (MA Khan et al: Thymoquinone, as an anticancer molecule: from basic research to clinical investigation. *Oncotarget* 2017 Aug 1: 8(31):51907-19; WM Yimer et al: *Nigella sativa* L. (black cumin): A promising natural remedy for wide range of illnesses. *Evid Based Complement Alternat Med* 2019:1528635)
- Frankincense—Anti-inflammatory, analgesic, anti-depressant, sedative.
- Garlic—Immune system, cancer, heart disease.
- Hyssop—Hyperglycemia, expectorant.
- Mint—Diarrhea, menstrual cramps, nausea, headaches.
- Mustard—Cancer.
- Myrrh—Anti-parasitic, anti-fungal, anti-bacterial.
- Saffron—Cancer, depression, weight loss.

Herbs, plants noted in the Quran. TibbeNabawi, Islamic prophetic healing. Current uses:

Arabic	English	Uses
Adas	Lentils	alkalize, digestive, heart health; immune system, blood sugar, helps weight control
Arak	Toothbrush tree	diabetes, headache, etc.
Basal	Onion	colds, fever, flu, diarrhea, etc.

Arabic	English	Uses
Henna/Hina	Henna	cosmetics, headache, increase memory, etc.
Inab	Grapes	80% wine, 7% raisins and vinegar – liver & lung disorders, brain, cancer
Kafor	Camphor	tetanus, TB, muscle relaxant
Khajoor	Date palm	asthma, health tonic, memory
Rehan	Sweet basil	fragrant, food; mild nervous disorders, TB, skin diseases
Rumman	Pomegranate	great medicinal value: anti-oxidant, anti-bacterial, anti-microbial; liver problems, TB
Soom	Garlic	infections, flu, colds, blood pressure
Treen	Figs	inflammation, infections

Nigella sativa (Black seed)—From fennel flower plant; no relation to common cumin. Extremely nutritious; considered the cure for all diseases; God's plant.

Note: History reveals lentils were consumed in the Near East 13,000 years ago. Most Americans (83%) seem to ignore the benefits of this high-protein food. Here's what one cup of lentils will provide in nutrition: 230 cal, 18g protein, 15g fiber, 3.5g sugar, 358g folate, 1mg manganese, 6.6mg iron, 356g phosphorus, 0.5mg copper, 731mg potassium, 71mg magnesium, 0.4mg vitamin B8, 2.5mg zinc, 1.3mg vitamin B5.

Modern medicine is no stranger to medicinal plants. More than 25% of the medicines commonly used today were derived from plants. Digitalis used for heart disease came from the foxglove. Penicillin was discovered in soil mold. Ephedrine, used to treat asthma, is made from ma huang, or ephedra, which has been used in China by billions of people for over 7,000 years.

Although herbal medicine has been used throughout the world for thousands of years, the AMA, FDA, and Big Pharma refuse to embrace or recognize them.

A friend of mine was being treated for prostate cancer by his doctor. His PSA numbers continued to be very high. I suggested an herbal formulation that has testimonials on how it has been effective in treating prostate cancer as well as restoring one's immune system when undergoing chemotherapy and radiation. After a couple months his PSA numbers went down to 7, the lowest since being under the care of his doctor. After continuing on the herbal formulation, his PSA went to 4+ in another 30 days. The doctors and nurses at the clinic were celebrating. My friend and his wife were in ecstasy. He finally told his doctor that he had been taking an herbal product. At that point, the doctor refused to continue having him as a patient if he continued on the herbs. I told him, he's your doctor. He knows your medical issues more than I do. My friend stopped taking the herbal products and continued with his doctor. He died three months later. I've seen cancer patients cured by supplements. However, most doctors will say, "The original cancer diagnosis was no doubt incorrect."

Read about (Google) the Canadian cancer nurse Rene Caisse and how she struggled with the Canadian and US medical associations.

I contacted at least a half-dozen Alzheimer Associations in the US concerning herbal/mineral products that had been used with Alzheimer patients. *Not one reply.* I was using a few supplements on my wife, for memory. I hoped to find other people with some experience in herbal/mineral products for AD. Zilch. At the time of this writing, there are a few herbal/mineral products being advertised on TV for improving memory and nourishing the brain.

Here's the typical reaction by medical doctors when sup-plements are mentioned. The situation involved another large government-funded study that found vitamin D deficiency can increase the risk of mental impairment up to 400%.

Medical doctors will warn their patients: "This does not mean taking supplements is a good idea."

A large study is under way to determine if taking supplements is safe and if they can help prevent a variety of diseases. Let's do another study. Let's pursue another grant. Surely, we need more data. We've got money to burn. There must be 30,000 studies on vitamin D. I would imagine that vitamin E has also racked up 30,000 studies. Years ago vitamin C surpassed its 50,000[th] study. What a waste of limited medical research funds. Appar-ently, there is a bottomless money pit when it comes to funding studies on supplements—trying to "scientifically" prove they are not effective. Could they possibly have another motive? Would you believe they have tried to developed synthetic vitamins? Why? So they can obtain patents and market their invention for ten times the price of the natural vitamin. With the synthetics (chemicals) we would be blessed with all their side effects. Then our doctors can prescribe another synthetic (drug) to reduce the side effects. When my mother-in-law died, her death certificate listed "toxicity" as cause of death—she was taking fourteen med-ications. Seven were to address the side effects of the other seven.

A recent editorial in the journal *Annals of Internal Medicine* (2014) by a group of MDs made this comment: "Enough is Enough: Stop Wasting Money on Vitamin and Mineral Supple-ments ... they have no clear benefit and may be harmful."

"National Health and Nutrition Survey"... More than 93% of US adults do not meet dietary intake recommendations of vita-mins D and E. Magnesium is lacking in 61%; 50% lack calcium and 43% lack vitamin C. These are the results of our "calorie-rich, nutrient-poor dietary pattern of Western populations." (Linus Pauling Institute Newsletter, Spring/Summer, 2014)

According to health authorities at Oregon State University, the Seattle Children's Hospital, Oakland Research Institute, Tufts University, and the Harvard School of Public Health, most people in the US do not meet all the guidelines for dietary intake of vitamins and minerals.

"It's naive to ignore the fact that most people have micronutrient inadequacies, and wrong to condemn a daily supplement that could cover these nutritional gaps" – Balz Frei, PhD, professor and director of the OSU Linus Pauling Institute.

If the nutritional approach is not sufficient for some people, what other choices are available? First, we must decide if our food products contain their proper minerals and vitamins. Can we trust organic food products? If they were grown in mineral-deficient soils, we could be at risk. If the organic food products contain GMOs, they may contain fewer minerals and vitamins. If we feel an illness like the flu or a cold coming on, do we reach for a drug or a supplement? A drug has a quick reaction...a few days or a week. The nature of a supplement is to prevent the illness; however, they take longer to have an effect...a few weeks or a month. With my high immune system, I prefer supplements to ward off an illness.

Our health goal should be to prevent an illness or disease, rather than becoming infected and relying on a medication and/or surgery for treatment.

The plan entitled The Rejuvenation of Senility prior to the 1970s may be the best option we have to prevent memory loss associated with Alzheimer's. At this writing, years of research and funding by Big Pharma has produced nothing. Not one of their 250-plus drugs for AD has passed Phase III Clinical Trials, after investing near $800 billion. Nothing has been accomplished to treat, reverse, or cure Alzheimer's.

With medicinal herbs being used for 5,000 years, I will start with those. In order to maintain and increase the life and mind of the human body, the "healers" drew upon the thousands of herbs that were being used. These were called natural medicines created by our Creator. One leading researcher at the University of Texas stated: "We've never had as much success with chemicals invented by man as we're having with plant extracts."

As Stephen Hawking stated: "All of our plants to sustain life have been created—it's up to man to find them."

Herbs for preserving and restoring youth have been investigated by researchers from England, France, and Russia. These herbs include ginseng, fo-ti-tieng, gotu kola, sarsaparilla, and damiana. Ginseng is the most famous and potent plant. It has been used by millions of Chinese for over 7,000 years as an aphrodisiac, rejuvenator, revitalizer, and cure-all for a variety of illnesses. If it is "snake oil"—as some doctors proclaim—why is it still in such demand?

- Ginseng—The Asians claim: It strengthens the heart, revitalizes the nervous system, increases hormone production, and stimulates cell growth and activity.
- Fo-ti-tieng—Grows in the tropical jungles of Asia. It was popularized by Chinese herbalist, Professor Li Chung Yun, also known as He-Shou-Wu (Fo-Ti). British, French, and Ceylonese researchers studied and had clinical tests on the "unknown Vitamin X" showed it had a rejuvenating effect on brain cells and endocrine glands. It stimulates the adrenal glands and helps detoxify the body. Prof. Li used this herb tea all his life – 256 years, outlived 24 wives.
- Gotu kola—Similar to fo-ti-tieng and ginseng. It has a marked energizing effect on the cells of the brain and a strengthening effect on the nerve functions. It is also used as a diuretic, a kidney stimulant and a blood purifier.

Records show that regular use of gotu kola increases longevity by strengthening the brain.

- Sarsaparilla—A tropical plant that grows in Honduras, Jamaica, and Mexico. The roots of the plant are used for making a tea. It's used for many conditions such as weakness and sexual impotence, and is also a known blood purifier. In several South American countries they manufacture testosterone tablets using sarsaparilla. Progesterone was also found in the roots of the plant.
- Damiana—Has been used by Indians in Mexico as an aphrodisiac and a general revitalizer for many centuries. The sexual virility largely determines man's youthfulness, health, vitality, and longevity.

The popular supplements that may reduce one's risk of Alzheimer's are:

- Acetyl-l-carnitine—A building block of proteins, naturally produced by the body.
- Bacopa monnieri—Memory recall.
- Choline bitartrate—Memory.
- Dandelion—Kidney and liver detox, inflammation.
- DMAE (dimethylaminoethanol)—Improves memory; small amounts produced in brain.
- Damiana leaf*
- Folic acid—Helps produce and maintain new cells.
- Forskolin—High blood pressure. ("Question: What are Natural Alternatives for Addressing Hypertension?" J. Pizzorno, ND, J. Katzinger, ND, *Vitamin Retailer*, August 2011)
- Siberian ginseng*
- Gotu kola, ginkgo biloba (optional)*

*covered on previous pages; **covered elsewhere in this chapter

- Grape seed extract—Slows down aging, increases cognitive function.
- He-Shou-Wu**
- Norwegian kelp **
- L-glutamine—Building blocks of protein.
- L-theanine—Reduces stress.
- L-tyrosine—helps brain produce neurotransmitters.
- Lecithin—Treatment of neurological disorders, Alzheimer's.
- Niacin (Vitamin B_3)—Boosts brain function.
- Periwinkle—Headaches, vertigo, poor memory—recorded uses from the 5th to the 15th century.
- Phenylalanine—Amino acid for central nervous system.
- Phosphatidylserine—Improves memory and brain function.
- Turmeric—Reduces inflammation.
- Una de gato (cat's claw)—Immune system, antioxidant, memory.
- Vitamin A, B_3, B_6, B_{12}, C, D_3, E **
- Zinc **

Do not let this list frighten you. All of us have different chemistry, and a supplement that works for me may not work for you. Blame it on our DNA. Also, many of these minerals and vitamins are in the food products we consume.

There are numerous supplement manufacturers whose medical scientists (PhDs in biochemistry and MDs) formulate products that contain a number of these herbs, minerals, and vitamins to support the brain, heart, kidneys, liver, etc.

I take a proprietary nerve formula to help support proper nerve function: it contains acetyl-l-carnitine, l-taurine, phosphatidylcholine, alpha-lipoic acid, and lecithin.

---

*covered on previous pages; **covered elsewhere in this chapter

On alternate months I take another proprietary product—Clear Thoughts—to help support my memory. It contains vitamin E, d-alpha tocopherol succinate and acetate, niacin, folic acid, vitamin B_{12}, zinc, l-glutamine, gotu kola, l-tyrosine, ginkgo biloba, phosphatidylserine, damiana leaf, and choline bitartrate.

There's another herbal formulation that I'm testing to see how it acts with my chemistry. Rainforest Treasure Tea is for mental clarity, physical immunity, and vitality. It contains: jatoba, which is high in antioxidants for immune support; una de gato, which regulates mind-body harmony; pau d'arco, which helps with immune and microbial balance; Quebra Pedra, which supports kidney and urinary health, and chuchuhuasi, an antioxidant for immune support.

As new formulations go through laboratory testing, they will become available on the market. Supplements are quite different from drugs. Since the majority are not patented, they do not receive huge funding for testing.

You may recall fen-phen, the "diet cocktail" from Wyeth that was popular in the 1990s. It was deadly. The FDA finally requested its withdrawal from the market in 1997. By 2004, Wyeth had paid out $13.1 billion (reserve of $16.6 billion). As of 2018, Wyeth was negotiating to settle all outstanding claims with up to $4 billion.

During the 1990s I was an MLM distributor for a small supplement firm in the US that had the most successful diet product on the market. They tried to have it tested (for FDA approval) with clinical trials at a prestigious West Coast university at a cost of $25 million. Yet they could not patent the product. The success of the product was due to an ingredient from China—ma huang (ephedra sinca, native to China, Mongolia, and Russia, and used for asthma). Although ma huang had been used in China since 5000 bc (also by Native Americans and Mormon pioneers), the FDA banned it. Apparently, it was too successful. An herb?

How could that be? The daily dosage for ma huang was listed as 25 mg by the FDA.

My daughter (BS, Nursing) had an asthma attack that almost took her life. Three doctors said they had done all they could for her with drugs. She could not lie down to rest. She slept sitting up. Finally, her husband called the PhDs (biochemists) who formulated an herbal diet capsule. They recommended a dosage of 300 mg per day, plus the addition of minerals for her heart muscles. In three days she was back to normal. By continuing with the drugs, she would have died. For the fen-phen story read *Dispensing with the Truth* by Alicia Mundy. "They" all knew the fen-phen diet cocktail was a killer. But "they" dragged their feet until an EKG technician in Fargo, ND, slammed her file on the desk of the cardiologists.

In 2011, a friend of my daughter became the victim of the "flesh-eating disease"—necrotizing fasciitis, often caused by *Vibrio vulnificus*. The infection is fatal in 12 to 20 hours with 30 to 40% fatality rates. She knew enough about the signs and symptoms to drive herself to the local hospital. She was also a person who had been taking many supplements (herbs, minerals, vitamins) to maintain her well-being for the previous 20 years. The coloring on her arm was spreading. With her temperature at 104, her organs began to shut down. They rushed her to a major hospital in Portland, which called in a doctor who was familiar with the disease. Her family brought in her stash of specific supplements for immune building, plus antibiotics. Sections of her arm were phasing from red to purple. The doctor (a specialist on the "flesh-eating disease") had her on their "high performance" drugs. Blood testing revealed no change. As the day passed, relatives were told she might not survive. They called her minister. To save her life, the doctor scheduled an operating room for amputating her arm. There was nothing more Western medicine could do. She felt sick, and her memory was fading. Finally, she lost all memory. After taking numerous supplements, receiving drug injections, and being connected to the monitor, her last blood draw indicated the infection had stopped and her white count was dropping. No need for amputating her arm—which may or may not have saved her life. A week in the hospital and the coloring in her arm improved. It took a couple months for the color of her arm to return to normal. Her doctor in charge said that anyone half her age would have died. She was 79.

Will "snake oil" perform its miracle on a youngster? My neighbor's daughter is living proof. She was born with the birth defect spina bifida, a neural tube disorder. Her defect was at a position on the spine where she was not paralyzed. However, she did not have control of her bladder and bowel. Her father knew a couple of scientists (PhDs in biochemistry) who formulated a remarkable new product that opened the eyes of many "non-believer" medical doctors. He called it "snake oil with scorpion venom as a chaser." Their proprietary product contained a bioflavonoid blend, grapefruit pectin, acerola fruit, milk thistle, plus EnriDole 3-C (indole-3-carbinol). Indole-3-carbinol had been researched for years. Studies were conducted by internationally famous research scientists and medical doctors as early as the mid-1950s in Czechoslovakia. The National Academy of Sciences, the *Journal of the National Cancer Institute*, Royal Society of Edinburgh, *Cancer Research*, and *Nutrition and Cancer* have all been involved in the studies. Her kidney damage was reversed. Various body parts were all normal. Her kidneys, which were weakened by spina bifida, were also working at a higher rate than when she was born. Her pediatric urologist was shocked. Her file made medical history on spina bifida, as 99.9% of all doctors will confirm that nerve function is not likely to improve in a child with spina bifida. After being on "super antioxidants" for a couple months, her kidneys were functioning with an 18% increase. As she grew older, I joked with her about being a "guinea pig" (at Children's Hospital in Seattle). She corrected me: "I'm a medical pioneer." Her medical godfather is the retired director of Children's Hospital, a gifted and talented Harvard MD who wrote the book on spina bifida. This medical pioneer lives in Seattle. She celebrated her 35th birthday in 2018. She also had her 30th surgery (first procedure of its type in the world) in 2017. In 2019 she received an award in neuroscience from the University of Washington Medical Center. Oh yes, she has faith in supplements.

In her early years as a patient at Children's Hospital, she met a young boy, Peter, who had cloacal exstrophy, a severe birth defect wherein much of his abdominal organs (bladder and intestines) was exposed. As a result his kidneys were working at 18%. His mother asked his urologist if it would be okay to start her son on these new ("snake oil") pills. In a few months his kidneys were working at 33%—a 183% increase. Peter's grandpa had emphysema that required him to carry an oxygen bottle at all times. After a few months on the super antioxidant, grandpa got rid of the oxygen bottle and began riding his bicycle. Not bad for what some doctors would call "snake oil."

A year ago, I was scheduled for surgery to remove an internal cyst in my abdomen. From the day I was in the doctor's office when the surgery date was set, I began a regimen of herbs to dissolve the cyst. Two herbs did their job at a cost of less than $30. The doctor was amazed, and I did not require the surgery.

For those readers who would like to see some evidence of anticipated problems with consumption of herbs, minerals, and vitamins, consider the list that notes the number of poisonings reported in *Townsend Letter for Doctors*.

The most popular herbs: ginseng, echinacea, dandelion, dong quai, astragalus, He-Shou-Wu, goldenseal, hawthorn.

The total number of poisoning deaths: zero.

The most popular vitamins and minerals: vitamin A, B, C, D, E and vitamin B-complex, iron, zinc, calcium, magnesium, and potassium.

The total number of poisoning deaths: zero.

The most popular pharmaceuticals: analgesics, antidepressants, antihistamines, antimicrobials, asthma therapies, cardiovascular drugs, cough and cold preparations, gastrointestinal preparations, hormones and hormone antagonists, anti-anxiety/anti-psychotics, and topicals.

The total number of poisoning deaths: 9,805. (The above data is from federal government statistics.)

I recall the rumor about people dying from consuming the herb hawthorn (berries) for improving cardiovascular health. We laughed when we learned the truth from the original source. The "people" who became ill, with a few dying, were a flock of starlings who consumed fermented hawthorn berries. They flew into large glass windows.

Herbs, minerals, vitamins, and their formulations will be listed as supplements in this chapter. (From the following sources: *Herbs in Your Life,* by James C. Adams (BS, M Ed, Ed S) 1996 Edition. *The Encyclopedia of Natural Remedies* by Louise Tunney, Master Herbalist, 1995 Edition. *Are You Confused* by Paavo Airola, (ND, PhD) 1971 edition.)

HERBS–SINGLE

- **Burdock**—the seeds contain arctigenin, which helps memory and is an anti-inflammatory.

- **Butcher's broom**—Known and used for over 2,000 years. It is an anti-inflammatory that lowers cholesterol and benefits the circulatory system.

- **Capsicum** (Cayenne)—Among other benefits, it helps reduce inflammation, normalizes blood pressure, helps control high cholesterol, and feeds cell structure of arteries.

- **Echinacea**—Among other benefits, it boosts the immune system, protects healthy cells from attack by viruses and bacteria, helps in the growth of healthy new cell tissue, and expels poisons and toxins.

- **Garlic**—An immune booster, antibacterial, and antiviral. It reduces blood pressure and cholesterol.

- **Ginger**—Helps lower cholesterol.

- **Siberian ginseng**—Considered the "King of Herbs"— Among numerous benefits, it has anti-aging qualities, helps with senility and dementia, improves mental alertness, energy, memory, and concentration.

- **Ginkgo** (Ginkgo biloba)—One of the oldest-living trees (150–200 million years). It has been used as a medicine for thousands of years, and in Europe since 1700s. It is now sold all over the world and is one of the top-selling herbs in the US. It increases blood flow to the brain. The following information on gingko biloba is from the Mayo Clinic: Effective for intermittent claudication (medical term for limping, impairment in walking), cerebral insufficiency (medical term for delirium, a syndrome of cerebral insufficiency) and Alzheimer's/multi-infarct dementia (medical term for when blood clots block small blood vessels in the brain and destroy brain tissue). However, the Mayo Clinic concludes that ginkgo is still under scientific investigation. Why? Ginkgo has been used by billions of people over the course of thousands of years. There have been thousands of tests that prove its effectiveness. Are they investigating the possibility of developing a synthetic ginkgo? After all, the plant cannot be patented. Look at all the money Big Pharma is leaving on the table.

» Note: Years ago, a statement by a food products company seemed like a joke. They wanted to place wording on their prune juice label that it was a laxative. FDA rejected their request without undergoing scientific clinical trials conducted by a certified laboratory. Legality trumps common sense.

- **Gotu kola**—Referred to as the "longevity and memory herb," it stimulates circulation to the brain. Gotu kola is one of the most important herbs in Ayurveda medicine of India. According to ancient records, the leaves of the gotu kola plant are part of the elephant's diet. Its habitat is the tropical swamps of Australia, India, Madagascar, Pakistan, South Africa, South America, and Sri Lanka. Gotu kola has been used for thousands of years for numerous health conditions, most recently, Alzheimer's. It is not recommended for people with high cholesterol or diabetes.

- **He Shou Wu**—Known in China as a youth preserver, it filters out toxins, and is good for the brain and memory.

- **Norwegian kelp**—Helps eliminate waste and toxic metals; contains approximately thirty trace and major minerals; strengthens brain tissue.

- **Lobelia**—A strong relaxant; aids in circulation.

- **Milk Thistle**—A liver cleanser used to detox the whole body.

- **Passionflower**—a pure and natural, mild sedative, very relaxing; helps with stress and anxiety.

- **Pau d'arco**—An "everything" herb; it has anti-tumor and anti-fungal properties, and is a powerful antibiotic, among other benefits.

- My favorite. With my chemistry, this natural antibiotic works better than a drug. On two occasions I was out of the country and got an abscessed tooth. After I mega-dosed on Pau d'arco for three days, the swelling and pain were gone. When I returned home 10 days later, my dentist took care of the problem. He was amazed. The herb worked faster than the usual drug.

- **Psyllium**—Helps lower cholesterol.

- **Suma**—Contains essential vitamins, minerals, and amino acids.

MINERALS

- **Boron**—A trace mineral. Deficiency may impair mental functioning and depress mental alertness. Apricots, prunes, and dried fruit are the best sources.

- **Calcium**—Essential for a healthy, functioning body; cannot be absorbed without vitamin D.

- **Chromium**—Vital for proper sugar metabolism.

- **Copper**—To produce enzymes needed to facilitate the production of energy and produce the important neurotransmitters epinephrine, norepinephrine, histamine, serotonin, and dopamine.

- **Iodine**—The thyroid gland uses iodine to produce two thyroid hormones, T3 and T4. Thyroid hormones regulate all functions of every cell.

- **Iron**—Supports brain development, immune function, and temperature regulation.

- **Magnesium**—Found in bones and muscles. It supports the formation of proteins and fatty acids, and also serves as a co-factor for more than 300 enzymes.

- **Manganese**—Required to produce connective tissues and bones. It also supports the production of sex hormones, the regulation of blood sugar, and the absorption of calcium.

- **Molybdenum**—Necessary for the production of enzymes that support chemical reactions in the body.

- **Potassium**—Helps maintain fluid balance in the body. It is also important for muscle growth and neuromuscular activity.

- **Selenium**—Combines with protein in the body to form selenoproteins that act as antioxidants, compounds that protect cells from damage caused by negatively charged particles.

- **Silicon**—Found in the blood, muscles, skin, nerves, nails, hair, connective tissue, and teeth. The pancreas is rich in silicon. Noted for its use in antiseptic action.

- **Zinc**—Promotes enzyme activity, supports immune function, and aids in wound healing, DNA synthesis, and cell division.

VITAMINS

- **Beta carotene**—Alpha carotene, beta carotene, genistein, lycopene, lutein, zeaxanthin, beta-cryptoxanthin. Deficiency may be a co-risk factor in Alzheimer's, allergies, arthritis, asthma, cancer, dementia, heart disease, low immune system, etc.

- **Complex**—B_1 (thiamine), B_2 (riboflavin), B_3 (niacin), B_5 (pantothenic acid), B_6 (pyridoxine), B_7 (biotin), B_9 (folic acid), B_{12} (cyanocobalamin), choline, and inositol. Deficiency may be a co-risk factor in Alzheimer's, asthma, arthritis, cancer, cardiovascular disease, depression, diabetes, neurological damage, etc. According to neurologists at Loyola University Medical Center, deficiency of thiamine can cause a fatal brain disorder.

- **Vitamin C**—Deficiency may be a co-risk factor in Alzheimer's disease, asthma, high cholesterol, heart disease, hypertension, low immune system, etc. A powerful antioxidant. Huge doses can protect us against any acute poisoning from virtually any source, according to Dr. W. J. McCormack, an authority on vitamin C.

- **Vitamin D**—Deficiency may contribute to mineral imbalance, osteoporosis, rickets, and tooth decay.

- **Vitamin E**—D-alpha-tocopherol succinate. Deficiency may be a co-risk factor in Alzheimer's disease, progression of Alzheimer's, asthma, cancer, diabetes, heart disease, low immune system, etc.

- **Vitamin K**—Cholecalciferol. Deficiency may be a co-risk factor in birth defects, depression, diabetes, mental impairment, high cholesterol, low immune system, etc.

"Vitamins E and B_{15}, pangamic acid, can help to protect us from slow poisoning by carbon monoxide, to which we are all subjected."– Paavo Airola, PhD, ND

OTHER SUPPLEMENTS

Omega-3 fatty acids containing EPA/DHA. The anti-inflammatory benefits of omega-3 are becoming apparent in studies on Alzheimer's, arthritis, cancer, and heart disease. (Gleaned from several hundred medical research papers, studies and articles by MDs, PhDs, and NDs)

In 2015, the market for brain health supplements was valued at $2.3 billion in the US. By the year 2024, this market is projected to reach $11 billion. These brain health supplements concentrate on stress reduction, improving alertness, and enhancing cognitive performance. Established in the late 2000s, AddNeuroMed Project is a European private/public consortium. Their efforts relate to the study and pursuit for novel biomarkers for Alzheimer's.

WHAT DIOXIN DOES TO OUR IMMUNE SYSTEM

Dioxin is one of the most potent synthetic chemical toxins that man has ever produced. It is developed by a chlorine bleaching process. Wood pulp fiber is bleached with dioxin. It is present in products we use every day, including toilet paper, sanitary napkins, tampons, paper towels, tissues, milk cartons, juice cartons, coffee filters, tea bags, paper plates and cups, packaging of TV dinners, certain foods—and the list goes on. Dioxin is also in our environment, in the air we breathe and the water we drink. It is suspected that immune suppression, liver disorders, cancer, and birth defects are caused by dioxin. Tampons are treated with dioxin. The bleaching process sensitizes the vagina, making it more vulnerable to infection. If a woman's immune system is low, toxic shock syndrome could develop.

The 2,4,5-T used to produce Agent Orange (AO) was contaminated with tetrachlorodibenzodioxin (TCDD), an extremely toxic dioxin compound. Agent Orange was manufactured by

Monsanto and Dow Chemical for the US Department of Defense. During the Vietnam War, between 1962 and 1971, the US military sprayed nearly 20 million gallons of material containing herbicides and defoliants mixed with jet fuel in Vietnam, and parts of Laos and Cambodia. The US government is now paying the Vietnamese government hundreds of millions of dollars to repair the damage we inflicted on their country (the soils) and the citizens with AO-related health problems. There could also be 200,000 US veterans eligible for compensation. Dioxin exposure is an environmental risk factor for ischemic heart disease (reduced blood supply), birth defects (their offspring), dementia, type-2 diabetes, lung cancer, and Parkinson's.

As far as I know, there is no medication that will reverse the chemical-dioxin damage that was inflicted upon the human body. I offered to work with Vietnam veterans and use supplements, primarily herbal formulations. Neither *The Oregonian* nor veteran organizations would give me one veteran's name and phone number. I could not blame them; there are too many scams in our society.

Finally, I met a couple from Vietnam living about ten blocks from my home. He was an officer in their Navy and his wife was a pharmacist. His immune system was in very bad condition. He could not spend much time outside doing yard work or gardening. He was weak and had severe allergies. I doubt if he was over 50. I put him on a mild herbal formulation. I checked the vents in their home to ensure they were clean. They were a mess. All of the vents were plugged with small scraps of wood and sawdust from construction. The building contractor must have been "a quart low" or maybe he just fell off a turnip truck. In a few months, the ex-Vietnamese Naval officer felt like a new man. After a year of taking supplements, he was almost back to normal and working in his garden. It's very difficult to cleanse chemicals from our body with another chemical.

OTHER SUBSTANCES

In 2003, Mark A. McDaniel, MD, and others reviewed double-blind placebo studies of several non-prescription compounds used as memory enhancers and treatments for age-related memory decline. (McDaniel MA et al. "Brain-specific" nutrients: a memory cure? *Nutrition* 2003 Nov-Dec; 19(11-12):957-75) Some of the compounds examined were phosphatidylserine (PS), phosphatidylcholine (PC), vinpocetine, acetyl-l-carnitine (ALC), and antioxidants (particularly vitamin E). In the review, McDaniel wrote (my paraphrase): For older adults with moderate cognitive impairment, PS produced modest increases in recall of word lists. PC was not proven effective. Vinpocetine at 30 mg/day to 60 mg/day appeared to have some benefit in increasing blood circulation and acting as an antioxidant. ALC appeared to reverse many age-associated deficits in cellular function, in part by increasing cellular energy (ATP—adenosine triphosphate) production. The basic science evidence supports the suggestion that age-associated accumulation of mitochondrial deficits due to oxidation damage is likely to be a major contribution to an organism aging. ALC is usually given in doses of 1 to 3 g/day. The inability to efficiently generate energy is one of the most consistent finding in aging cells. The cells of the brain and heart require the largest amounts of energy to work efficiently.

Co-enzyme Q10 and alpha-lipoic acid act as antioxidants and improve efficiency of the pathways in seniors. There is increasing evidence that CoQ10 increases brain and cognitive function through these mechanisms.

Alpha glycerylphosphorylcholine (A-GPC) is water soluble, crosses the blood-brain barrier, and has been found to improve cognition in individuals with AD. It has also been found to increase growth hormone production in the pituitary gland and aid in brain recovery from strokes or anesthesia. In the trials, an average of 1,200 mg/day was used in divided doses. More than

95% of those in the trials had positive responses to GPC. A-GPC is considered one of the most effective brain nutrients in the world. (McDaniel MA et al. "Brain-specific" nutrients: a memory cure? *Nutrition* 2003 Nov-Dec; 19(11-12):957-75)

Adequate intake of EFAs and reduction of saturated fat intake benefit seniors by reducing the risk of atherosclerosis, inhibiting platelet aggregation, and reducing abnormal heart rhythms that increase the risk of strokes. Foods that contain the precursors for the essential fatty acid omega-3 include flax, walnuts, soy, pumpkin, and algae.

"In order for the body to take the linolenic acid in these foods and convert it to omega-3, enzymatic pathways must have adequate vitamins B_3, B_6 and C, as well as zinc and magnesium. Cold-water fish and algae have high concentrations of the omega-3 docosahexaenoic acid (DHA)." (Senior Health: "Cognitive Function to Seniors" by Wendy Arthur, MD, *Vitamin Retailer*, 54-55, May 2005)

CHAPTER 12

DRUGS—PRESCRIPTION MEDICATIONS

Numerous websites reveal some startling information concerning Big Pharma, the pharmaceutical industry in the United States:

"The puzzling rise and fall of a promising Alzheimer's drug." (Source: PubMed Central Journal List, 2010)

"Why So Few Drugs for Alzheimer's Disease? Are Methods Failing Drugs?" (Source: Aristea Translational Medicine Corporation and Drug Design & Development Section, Laboratory of Neurosciences, Intramural Research Program, National Institute of Aging, National Institutes of Health, 2008)

To an applied research engineer, this is extremely disturbing, based on the fact that the current medications prescribed for Alzheimer's patients in the US were developed by foreign medical laboratories, not Big Pharma.

Medical research groups are questioning their methodology to find the cause of Alzheimer's. "Does Alzheimer's cause the amyloid-B (AB) peptides in the brain, or are they the result of Alzheimer's?"

Are the medical research scientists for Alzheimer's drugs following the same methodology as the medical research scientists who researched HIV/AIDS?

Note: The US funding for HIV/AIDS was $32 billion in FY 2017–2018 (requested). Domestic care and treatment, $20.7 billion; global, $5.4 billion; domestic cash and housing assistance (SSI & SSDI), $3.1 billion; domestic research (NIH), $2.2 billion, and domestic prevention, $700 million. The seven-year average 2012–2018, was $31.09 billion per year. In 2015 there were 36.7 million people living with HIV. Thirty-five million have died since the 1980s. Some treatments require a four-drug cocktail. In 2016, Gilead's sales were $12.9 billion for *one* HIV/AIDS drug. In 2015, those sales were $11.1 billion. This is only for the treatment to stay alive. It's prescribed until the end of life. Big Pharma has yet to find a cure. With sales of more than $10 billion a year to *treat* HIV, where's the incentive to find a cure? The current, numerous HIV/AIDS drugs have a current MSRP (manufacturer's suggested retail price) of $550 to $3,800 for 30 tablets.

Funding for HIV research within the Department of Health and Human Services in FY 2001 was $9.2 billion, predominately in the ethnic and racial minority community. The US has become the greatest funding source of the global response to HIV (source: AVERT). Nations with the highest percentage of adults with HIV are Swaziland, Botswana, Lesotho (26–23.3%). The US average is 0.30%. Bosnia is lowest at 0.009%.

The galantamine drug for treating Alzheimer's in the early 2000s had a MSRP of more than $500 for 30 tablets. I found it ineffective for my wife.

Medical scientists have known of AD for over 100 years. In reviewing the efforts by research groups in finding treatments for AD and possibly the cure, or the reversal, it seems like they are tossing darts. When medical science is still working on improving detection/diagnosis, they seem to be admitting current diagnosis is questionable or unsound. Before medical science can solve the Alzheimer's disease problem, it must locate and define its cause or causes.

Hope in a pill? A recent study has shown that the risk of developing AD may be reduced as much as 60% by long-term use—over two years—of nonsteroidal anti-inflammatory drugs (NSAIDs). Shorter usage of these drugs, ibuprofen, for example, could reduce the risk by as much as 35%, according to researchers from Johns Hopkins University and the National Institute on Aging. A regimen of low-dose (baby aspirin, 80 mg) aspirin may reduce plaques in the brain, which will reduce Alzheimer's disease pathology and protect memory, according to Kalipada Pahan, a neurological researcher at Rush University Medical Center.

You may recall that medical scientists have advised us to take a low-dose aspirin to prevent and manage heart disease and stroke since the 1970s. Doctors suggested taking a 325 mg aspirin in the event a person was having a heart attack. Current studies indicate that medical advice on taking low-dose aspirin to prevent heart attacks has been rescinded. Which group of medical scientists should we believe? Note: The chronic use of some NSAIDs is associated with ulcer and kidney disease. It seems to me that more clinical trials are required.

University of Kentucky researchers report that small strokes in strategic regions of the brain may greatly increase the risk of developing the overt symptoms of AD. This study provides hope that treatments and prevention strategies now used for strokes and other diseases such as atherosclerosis may prove helpful in treating some people with AD. ("News From The World Of Medicine"—All About Alzheimer's—I. Hope in a Pill? *Los Angeles Times*; II. A Stroke, Reuters, 2005)

An experimental vaccine has been developed that seems to be able to prevent two proteins (beta amyloid and tau) from occurring in the brains of animals. These are the two proteins found in the brain of AD patients after death.

Recent speculation about the cause of AD implicates insulin. Researchers at Rhode Island Hospital and Brown University Medical School have found that insulin concentrations in the brain drop dramatically in early AD and continue to fall as the disease progresses. They suggest that this may contribute to the cell death and neurofibrillary tangles characteristic of AD. Another hallmark of AD—low levels of a substance called acetyl-choline— also is directly linked to loss of insulin, all of which suggests that AD may be a form of diabetes. This opens up promising new possibilities in solving the enigma of AD. ("What You Need To Know Now" by Dr. Isadore Rosenfeld, *Parade*, January 15, 2006)

Maybe medical scientists will be urged to take that other fork in the road, try a new avenue, and consider alternative medicine—herbal, mineral, vitamin formulations in supplements. Maybe these products could be part of the solution required to prevent Alzheimer's.

"No novel agent, since approval of memantine in 2002 has successfully completed Phase III clinical trials"– PubMed.

Natural products such as herbs and minerals are not patentable, except in rare situations. The snowdrop bulb, which has been used for a century in Europe for enhancing memory, has been synthesized into the drug galantamine, one of the popular drugs for AD. Therefore, when a natural product is synthesized it becomes a patentable drug with millions, if not billions, of dollars of revenue awaiting. However, with the drugs, we are prone to side effects that have been known to cause death.

Currently, there must be a couple dozen drugs approved by FDA that are the subject of class action lawsuits. The pharmaceutical company that produces Avandia has set aside $6 billion to cover lawsuits. The lawsuit claims 83,000 heart attacks could have been the result of taking Avandia.

Following are the pharmaceutical drugs approved by FDA for Alzheimer's. (National Institute on Aging, US National Institutes of Health)

- Cognex (tacrine)—Approved in 1993 for mild to moderate AD; developed at the University of Sydney. It was withdrawn from use in 2013 for safety reasons.
- Aricept (donepezil)—Approved in 1996 for all stages of AD; developed by Eisai of Japan, marketed by Pfizer.
- Exelon (rivastigmine)—Approved in 2000 for all stages of AD; first skin patch for AD. Developed at the Department of Pharmacology at Hebrew University of Jerusalem.
- Razadyne (galantamine)—Approved in 2001 for mild to moderate AD. Developed by the Soviet Union and Russia between 1971 and 1993.
- Galantamine, Nivalin, Reminyl, Razadyne ER, Lycoremine—Manufactured synthetically or from the bulbs and flowers of Galanthus caucasicus (snowdrop). Usage as a modern medicine began in the Soviet Union in the 1950s. The active ingredient was extracted, identified, and studied by Soviet pharmacologists. The work of Mashkovsky and Kruglikova-Lvova was the first published work that demonstrated the acetylcholinesterase (AChE)-inhibiting properties of galantamine.
- Namenda, Ebixa (memantine)—Approved in 2003 for moderate to severe AD; researched and developed at University of Aberdeen, Scotland.
- *Dimebon (latrepirdine)—Antihistamine drug filed in Russia in 1963, published in 1985; repurposed (off-label) by Medivation for AD in 1997; US and Russian patents; potential for next drug approved for AD. (Published in

*not approved by FDA

Behavior Pharmacology, 2007; *Lancet,* 2008; *Neurology,* 2008; Pfizer licensed; Phase III Clinical Trials failed in 2011)

- *Enbrel (etanercept)—A biologic drug approved for arthritis, repurposed for AD.
  » Note: "Pfizer had clues arthritis drug may prevent Alzheimer's"—article by Christopher Rowland of the *Washington Post,* published in *The Oregonian,* June 16, 2019.
- *Minipress (prazosin)—A drug used to treat high blood pressure, repurposed for AD; research at Oregon Health Sciences University, 2007; research at University of Washington ADRC, 2010; NIH, NIA, VA, clinical trials May 2010; verified November 2013; effective for behavioral symptoms; estimated completion date, July 2015. Trials of 9 and 12 weeks with 24 patients. Improvement in behavior found. A larger trial of 200 patients is planned.
- *Gantenerumab—Hoffman-La Roche (Switzerland)— Estimated study completion date, 2020.
- *Solanezumab—Eli Lilly—Phase III trials failed in summer of 2013.
- *Immunotherapy—The treatment of disease by inducing, enhancing, or suppressing an immune response.
- *Beta-Secretase Inhibitor—A prime drug target for the levels of amyloid beta.
- *Anti-Amyloid Antibody Crenezumab—Developed by Swiss-based biopharmaceutical company AC Immune; licensed to Genentech, Inc. (Roche) in 2006. First trials in Medellin, Colombia, revealed no benefit to AD patients. However, AD appears at age 45 in this family of 300. New trials began in 2013 on the first prevention trial to be completed by 2020.

---

*not approved by FDA

- *Bapineuzumab—Johnson & Johnson—Phase III trials failed in summer of 2013.
- *Phenserine—developed by Axonyx, US, NIH technology, next generation acetylcholinesterase (AChE) inhibitor; licensed to QR Pharma, a start-up; it failed in Phase III trials in 2009.
- *Posiphen—developed by Axonyx, Inc., US, and NIH; related to Phenserine; new trials pending.
- *Metrifonate—Manufactured by Bayer; proposed for AD; approved by FDA; no longer in development; Phase III trials failed.
- *Flurizan (tarenflurbil)—Years of trials by Myriad Genetics concluded in 2008; discontinued when Phase III trials failed. Sold to Lundbeck in Copenhagen (manufacturer of memantine, Namenda, and Ebixa; developed at University of Aberdeen, Scotland).
- *Tramiprosate, Alzhamed, Vivimind—Developed by Neurochem (now Bellus Health, Inc.) of Laval, Quebec, Canada, "to hinder the formation of amyloid plaque." After $250 million and fifteen years, the Phase III Clinical Trials failed. Bellus is investigating Tramiprosate as a natural product (not patentable and not required by the FDA to undergo clinical testing) for AD.
- *Rosiglitazone (GlaxoSmithKline)—Phase III clinical trials, 2007–2014 complete; no study results.
- *Anipryl (selegiline)—developed at Semmelweis University in Budapest; limited trials at University of Oxford, UK, 2003; no benefit for AD patients shown.
- *Aducanumab—a treatment for AD that targets the beta amyloid. Neurimmune Therapeutics AG is a biopharmaceutical company in Switzerland. A research team at

---

*not approved by FDA

the Univdersity of Zurich discovered the drug. Biogen co-develops the drug with Eisai of Japan (donepezil— brand name Aricept was developed by Eisai in 1983 and approved by FDA in 1996). The Phase II study of the drug was reported in March 2015. The Phase III clinical trials halted after it did not meet the primary end point of the drug in March 2019 and restarted in October 2019. Note the recent article ("Experts split over Alzheimer's drug", by Marylynn Marchione, Associated Press, as reported in *The Oregonian*, December 8, 2019). This is a promising AD drug that reveals the cooperation of three countries striving to satisfy a global market.

Big Pharma has taken a big hit in their vault. Along with a couple dozen class action lawsuits in the billions of dollars, add to that their failures to cure with the AIDs and Alzheimer's drugs in research, plus the lost revenue from expired patents. Big Pharma must be bleeding like a stuck hog.

Since 2009, a dozen of their billion-dollar drug patents have expired—Lipitor: $6.4 billion; Actos: $2.6 billion; Flomax: $1.3 billion; Aricept: $1.2 billion, and others, for a total of $27.8 billion. From the "fake news" media, I understand Big Pharma has put their muscle on Congress to extend their expired patents to prevent the manufacturing of generic drugs. That would be in violation of US patent laws.

With alligators up to their neck, that could explain why the Big Three—AMA, Big Pharma and FDA—have been hammering the supplement industry with false accusations.

Anavex Life Sciences Corporation, founded in New York in 2004, is a clinical stage biopharmaceutical company engaged in the development of novel drug candidates to treat Alzheimer's,

*not approved by FDA

CNS diseases, and various types of cancer, which have significant unmet medical needs. Anavex 2-73, their new drug candidate developed to treat AD, has undergone an initial Phase I human clinical trial. It was well tolerated in doses up to 55 mg. Pre-clinical studies indicate that Anavex 2-73 demonstrates anti- amnesic and neuroprotective properties. After briefing myself on their research in the past few years, I'm of the opinion that Anavex LSC may be on the right path to a drug that could reverse memory loss in Alzheimer's victims. A synergistic effect has been observed between Anavex 2-73 and Aricept. The combined drugs—called Anavex Plus—produced up to 80% greater reversal of memory loss in AD models versus when the drugs were used individually. A human trial was conducted at a hospital in Victoria, Australia, with results in 38 days. The same type of trial with Aricept took six months, with its results remaining useful. Let's keep our fingers crossed.

Lithium is found in vegetables, nuts, seeds, grains, and fish as well as some meat and dairy products. Lithium orotate is a specific form of lithium salts that offers the benefits of standard lithium without the harmful side effects. In minimal doses, lithium appears to have medically important and positive impacts on mental health.

Stem cell therapy for Alzheimer's recruiting is under way with a project of Longeveron of Miami, Florida. An interesting program to follow...I tried, but could not find the location of the testing. Mexico? Until I could find out any solid medical information, I will place this program on hold.

There's a medical group investigating the prospect of a "brain pacemaker" for Alzheimer patients. This could be promising. Pacemaker technology for the heart is quite common. My neighbor had a new heart pacemaker installed when she was 83. Her old device was about ten years old. The total cost of the new pacemaker, including the operation and her stay in the hospital, cost around $300,000 before all the patient "discounts." I imagine the initial cost for a "brain pacemaker" would have a price of at least $500,000. But would it improve the life of an Alzheimer's patient in the late stages of AD? Could they live alone? It could be promising.

The Journal of Neural Engineering (R Hampson et al, "Developing a hippocampal neural prosthetic to facilitate human memory encoding and recall," June 2019; 15(3):036014) reports on an interesting approach, but there is not enough data for me to even estimate an opinion.

The brain is a very delicate and vital organ of the human body. Take care of it and try not to abuse it. How many of us do? We bump into things and get a knot on our head. We play violent sports and take hits that can't be reversed.

You may not be able to plan for the day you are diagnosed with Alzheimer's, but you can plan for the day a loved one becomes a victim. You may be faced with a dilemma if you suspect that a family member may be in the early stage of Alzheimer's. If they are diagnosed and a medical doctor confirms the patient is in the early stages of AD, your life will change. Once the patient has been diagnosed with AD, you must begin the process of preparing for the bumpy road ahead. It is not an easy task, but if you are prepared, the road will be smoother. It can be navigated. I would suggest buying a journal for writing your notes. List the items that are most important for the care of your loved one. Don't wait until they have been diagnosed. Then it's a game of catch-up. You don't need the added stress. Also, you may want to begin a diary of daily or weekly observations if deemed necessary. Examples: If they lost their keys, it may not be too serious. Do they have a location for their keys? A hook in cupboard, a dish by the door to garage or on the night stand? Establish a common location. Did they forget an appointment? Most dentists and MDs, as well as veterinarians, call prior to an appointment as a reminder. Did they mark their calendar?

CONCLUSIONS

- "A public health approach to dementia could prevent up to 30% of worldwide dementia cases over the next twenty years. Brain health is commonly attributed to 70% lifestyle and 30% genetics." (Krystal L. Culler,et al. Published in June 2017– "Preventing Cognitive Decline and Dementia: A Way Forward." National Academies of Sciences, Engineering and Medicine.)

- Cognitive training; blood pressure management; increasing physical activity. (Published online in July 2017 – Prevention is Better Than a Cure–*Dementia Prevention, Intervention and Care*)

- Report by *Lancet* Commission: Co-risk factors leading to dementia/Alzheimer's: education; midlife hypertension; midlife obesity; hearing loss; depression; higher blood glucose levels; lack of physical activity; smoking, and social isolation.

- Launched in 2015, the Global Brain Health Institute, located at the University of California in San Francisco and Trinity College in Dublin, is a leader in protecting the world's aging population from threats to brain health. The Atlantic Fellows for Equity in Brain Health, based at GBHI, provides innovative training, networking, and support to emerging leaders. Connect with the GBHI at www.gbhi.org.

- The Global Council on Brain Health offers evidence-based recommendations for people to consider adopting into their daily lives. A collaborative of AARP, the council consists of scientists, health professionals, scholars, and policy experts from around the world working in broad areas of brain health. To date, the council has published reports on the following brain health topics: nutrition and brain health, cognitively stimulating activities, social engagement and brain health, sleep and brain health, and physical activity and brain health. For references, view this article at www.TodaysGeriatricMedicine.com

The following suggestions culled from numerous health books are designed to reduce one's risk of becoming a victim of AD. *(Note: We do not diagnose or prescribe.)* With all this data to absorb in such little time, consider the following recommendations based on your age group:

Under 30 years of age:
- Engage in a good exercise workout routine.
- Establish good eating habits with emphasis on fish, fruits, grains, nuts, poultry, seeds, vegetables.
- Take the minimum daily allowance of vitamins and minerals to make up for what you do not consume in food.
- Herbal supplements may include items to boost immune system and memory.
- Begin a whole body detox/cleanse routine monthly or quarterly.

Under 40 years of age:
- Continue with previous recommendations.
- Ensure your weight is under control.
- Add herbal products for memory (brain food).

Under 50 years of age:
- Continue with previous recommendations.
- Ensure your immune system is at its peak.
- Review your supplements and nutrition to ensure your well-being.
- Review your exercise routine with a health professional.

Under 60 years of age:
- Continue with previous recommendations.
- Consider annual medical checkup.
- Ensure your blood pressure is in the proper range, your cholesterol is around 200 or less, and your weight is in control for your age. Limit your salt intake to reduce hypertension.
  - » Note: there was a super blood pressure supplement that was banned for importation to the US in the 1990s. There were no side effects, such as possible liver and kidney damage. The formula was over 1,000 years old. It was formulated by Ibn Sina (Avicenna), the Islamic philosopher who was born in ad 980.

Over 60 years of age:
- Continue with all previous recommendations (for caregivers as well as for reducing risks).

Co-risk factors contributing to Alzheimer's
One risk is our potable drinking water. Municipal water systems can contain heavy metals including aluminum and lead, as well as chlorine and fluoride. To reduce risk, install a water filter. Quality filters can be purchased for around $150 and up.

Other risks are our environment, our atmosphere, and the air we breathe. To reduce our risk, consider a whole body detox with juice of lemon or a cleanse tea formulation to cleanse the liver, kidneys, and blood.

Don't purchase consumer products that are considered co-risk factors.

Consult your doctor and try to reduce your dependency on prescription drugs that increase your risk of AD.

Alcohol addiction—Until you reduce your consumption of alcohol to that of moderate or less, cleanse your liver with the herb milk thistle.

Drug addiction—Get help to reduce your dependency on street drugs and opiates. It can be done through supplements (herbs, minerals, vitamins) and determination.

Changeable risks can be reduced by exercise, family, nutrition, rest/sleep, social activity, supplements, and work environment.

Unchangeable risks are conditions that are beyond our control and we cannot change. They include our water (unless we filter), and our atmosphere (air filters in our home will help). We also can reduce our exposure to the co-risk factors.

CHAPTER 13

SUGGESTED EXERCISE (PHYSICAL AND MENTAL)

"It is exercise alone that supports the spirits, and keeps the mind in vigour."

– Marcus Tullius Cicero (January 106 bc–
December 43 bc), Roman lawyer, orator,
philosopher, statesman, writer

A heart attack put me in the hospital at the age of 37. My father suffered his first heart attack at 56. He died within 24 hours. Was this my time? I was lucky. It was a mere warning, and caused no damage. As a manufacturing engineer working with defense contractors, high stress was included in my job description. To add insult to injury, my first day home from the hospital almost gave me a stroke. My boss, the general manager, came to my home to inform me I had been terminated. The president of the firm did not want the liability of having an *invalid* on his payroll. So much for business ethics. As their sales engineer, I had wrapped up the largest contract in the history of the company with Boeing on the Minuteman Missile System. So much for gratitude.

Being out of a job, I concentrated on my body. I began an exercise regimen. When I was in the military, our company had a strict exercise routine—the "daily dozen." When I left the military, I was in great physical condition: 208 pounds at six foot, with a 30-inch waist. I passed the West Point physical test. Fifteen years later, I weighed 210 pounds and my waist was 34 inches. This came about by not following an exercise routine, other than salmon fishing, fly fishing, deer hunting, lawn mowing—light stuff. A daily jogging regimen brought me down to 175 pounds within a year. Because my ankles were weak (I broken them playing high school football), my ankle problems returned. My doctor advised me to give up jogging. He said it was bad for my back, with my type of frame. Years later, without a strict diet, my weight varies from 190 to 200 pounds. Through exercise and diet, I will reach my goal of 185.

After my wife's heart surgery (a single bypass due to a blood clot), we began our brisk walking routine. It was a brisk walk in our neighborhood, which included one long hill of five blocks. At least six days a week, we walked for 30 minutes, rain or shine. We met young people walking down the hill, decked out in the latest, trendy shoes, and designer sweats. Strange, they never followed through with their plan. Within a month, we never saw them again. I do hope they continued their walking routine in a gym or mall. For over 15 years, we maintained our walking routine. At rest, my heart rate decreased from the mid-60s to the mid-50s in a few months after beginning this regimen.

Note: Make sure you have a great pair of shoes. I had an Adidas trainer review my "test walk" when I got back into my brisk walking regimen. It was a warm day and my test walk was a brisk 3.5 miles. I came through with a bit of sweat, a normal pulse rate, but my feet were killing me. I was wearing a pair of worn out 10-year-old "Brand X" shoes. Slipping into the proper pair of Adidas was akin to walking on a cloud. My feet and legs thanked me.

Seattle researchers found that older adults who exercised three or more times a week lowered their risk of developing AD compared to those who exercised much less. (The report of Dr. Eric B. Larson from the Group Health Cooperative was published in the January 17, 2006, issue of the *Annals of Internal Medicine*.)

Exercise increases blood flow to the brain and promotes the growth of new brain cells. Dr. Carl Cotman and his team at the University of California-Irvine, found that exercise activates the production of a protein called brain-derived neurotrophic factor, or BDNF, which helps support the growth of existing brain cells and the development of new ones. As we age, BDNF levels decrease. Certain types of exercise, such as aerobic, will counteract these declines in BDNF.

If your budget will tolerate the expense, join a fitness center or gym where you can be monitored by a health professional. For the rest of us, establish an exercise routine in your apartment or home. Check with your doctors for their recommendations on a group of exercise types. I exercise in my home and use a stationary bicycle. It's always advisable to go through a stretching routine to reduce the shock to your muscles. When I'm in my lounge chair watching TV or reading, I have an exercise that keeps my leg and hip joints flexible. I bring my knees up as far as I can, one at a time, while flexing my ankle. I do about twenty repetitions every 60 minutes. I try not to watch TV more than one hour at one sitting.

Fast healing is a plus for older adults who exercise. Studies show that wound-healing time is greatly reduced through exercise, which also reduces the chance of infection. (A study by Charles Emery, a psychology professor at Ohio State University, centered on bike pedaling, jogging, brisk walking, and strength training.)

Exercise … sweat, exercise … sweat. Most health professionals suggest at least 15 minutes of exercise to work up a sweat. Anything less than fifteen minutes is not worth the effort. When our body sweats, we are detoxing our body of toxins through our pores. It is a necessity for a healthy life and well-being.

The graceful body movements of tai chi are recommended for everyone, especially seniors, to reduce their risk of dementia. Tai chi is good for improving balance, relieving stress, and combating fatigue. The gentle exercise also builds strength, strengthens the lower body, improves posture, and promotes flexibility. Researchers at Beijing University and Harvard Medical School focused on how tai chi helped people with medical problems. Of 507 studies, 94.1% found positive effects from practicing tai chi.

Michael Valenzuela of the School of Psychiatry, University of New South Wales, Australia, encourages memory-based exercises to reduce dementia by over 40%. Brain exercises keep the mind agile and active. Over the years, we have created a database in our brain. We know the birthdays and anniversaries of our family members, relatives, and close friends. In old movies we recognize Gina Lollobrigida, Paul Newman, Kim Novak, Marlon Brando, and Frank Sinatra. While listening to music, we recognize Brubeck, Ella, Shearing, Miles, Willie, Johnny, and a host of others.

Music has been part of my life since I can recall. As a tenor in my youth, I was the community entertainment at potlucks and dances. To this day, I listen to music most of the day, while reading, writing, gardening, and relaxing. Keeping time to the music by tapping your heels and toes is great for circulation in one's legs. As he is a jazz trumpeter, my son-in-law's favorite musician is Miles Davis. We attended a concert by Wynton Marsalis and the Lincoln Center Jazz Orchestra. It was a tribute to Duke Ellington. While listening to those talented and gifted musicians, one's emotions erupt. As we were keeping time to the music with our body movements, other concert patrons sitting around us gave us the stink eye, as if it was a sin to appreciate great music.

There is limited medical research concerning music as a prevention of AD. I was quite surprised to see data on the internet that questioned "could music cause AD?" As engineers, our discipline is to create; we favor prevention. There are other disciplines that favor treatment, which has a higher price tag. "When words fail, music provides a way" is a phrase used by numerous AD groups. Studies have reported physical, cognitive, and psychological benefits with music and dance therapy. (*Science Digest*) The Dutch information and analytics company Elsevier is a good source for more data on this subject.

My investigative mind forced me into finding more data to support the therapy of music to prevent and/or delay becoming a victim of AD. I searched the internet for the number of famous people who were AD victims. Of the first 150 people in the US I found, the majority were authors, singers, and film and TV stars, with politicians and sports figures being third in my unscientific probe. As I suspected, instrumentalists were last—jazz musicians. Glenn Campbell (1936–2017) was an American actor, guitarist, singer, songwriter, and TV host. George Russell (1923–2009) was an American arranger, composer, jazz pianist, and theorist. Herb Ellis (1921–2010) was an American jazz guitarist. They were the only instrumentalists to have AD out of 150 famous people.

Several years ago, through a writer friend of mine, I met Lorin Hollander, an American classical concert pianist who was called "the leading pianist of his generation" by a *New York Times* critic. Hollander introduced specific music to hard-core inmates at correctional institutes in the US. It decreased their tendency toward violence while in confinement. It may never become standard therapy for inmates, but time will tell. It's worth more study. The Institute for Music and Neurological Function recognized Lorin

Hollander with the 2003 "Music Has Power Award" for his advocacy of music and healing.

If we are good in math, we can reconcile our bank accounts without a calculator. By keeping our brain active, our memory bank does not decrease as rapidly as we age. By stimulating brain activity, we increase blood circulation and activate sections of the brain.

One of the greatest stories I can recall concerning the brain was about an American GI who was a prisoner of war during the Vietnam War. To maintain his sanity, he designed and built a house *in his mind*. The Viet Cong tried to mess up his mind, but he used his brain to survive. He imagined the design detail of each room. His brain provided the picture of the completed house through the construction phase. By doing so, his brain activity kept him active and wanting to live through his ordeal in a Viet Cong prison.

Crossword puzzles are great for stimulating the brain. For the higher brain stimulation, take up a new sport, learn a new language, take music lessons, return to a college or university and sign up for a class in ethics or politics—just kidding. Try courses in the arts and crafts. While I was an engineering student, my adviser suggested I take some courses that were not engineering oriented. I took a term of geology, which became so interesting that I took two more and almost changed my major to petroleum engineering. I find learning something new very exciting. Actually, cruising the internet is a great brain exercise. Research a famous person or a historical event; take a picture tour of Spain. They are all great brain exercises.

As a society, we shell out around $60 billion a year, as close as I can count, to keep our bodies in great shape. We try to lose weight, next is picture-perfect teeth with a Colgate smile, hair styling and tinting, then the nip and tuck of our body parts through gifted and talented cosmetic surgeons. But how much do we invest to improve our brain?

We actually torment and terrorize our brain with too much

booze, too many medications, street drugs, nicotine, the wrong type of foods, and whatever we can find to make us feel good. Eventually, all of our "sins" are transferred to our children, who emulate us and become the future of our society. As the older generation, we should be setting examples. Most of my friends during the early school years (grade and high school) considered me as being "sheltered." They envied me for my parents. My mother and my father were my role models. My mother never smoked or drank alcohol. Being a diabetic (from age 35 to 56), my father drank very little alcohol. I enjoyed my first small glass of beer with my father when I was 14. At Christmas holidays we enjoyed a Tom and Jerry. I could drink a beer and a mixed drink at home with family from the age of 16. Of course, there were times when I drank too much at a "beer party." I was not a choir boy. My father smoked cigarettes until he was 46, when his first granddaughter was born.

As we grow older, each generation adds more data to our "family database" where we store names, phone numbers, addresses, and the "life story" of each child and grandchild. Eventually, our brain becomes overloaded. As I get older, I try not to store irrelevant data in my brain. I also maintain my daily diary. Some days I merely make a note of the weather. I have saved my daily diaries from when I was in my mid-30s.

Exercising the mind at any age may stimulate brain growth and help maintain robust mental function throughout life.

In 2002, a large clinical trial funded partly by the National Institute on Aging revealed the benefits of more targeted mental training. A 5- to 6-week course in problem solving or speedy information handling yielded improvements that on average would have reversed 7 to 14 years of cognitive decline. Other studies indicate that the human brain can regenerate.

A Swedish analysis of 13 population studies in June 2004 linked improved cognitive function and reduced cognitive decline with mental stimulation from leisure activities.

To hone your brain, try experimenting with mnemonics, a technique that uses associations to link information. (For example, the acronym ROY G. BIV helps you remember the colors of the rainbow.) When I was working in Mobil and Chevron service stations, I remembered customers by their cars. To this day I can recall the names of men who owned Buicks, Cadillacs, Fords, etc.

When I'm stuck in traffic, I don't get upset. I glance at all the license plates in my view and add the numbers in my head. I play numbers games. While singing in church or wherever I see the lyrics, I form a picture in my mind of the words ... river, meadow, tree, table, whatever. Being ADD, I can multitask, which is not good for my brain, according to current medical scientists.

The University of Texas at Austin offers mnemonics at www.utexas.edu/student/utlc/makinggrade/mnemonic. It's important to cultivate ongoing, enjoyable mental pursuits, each of which may be especially useful for specific skills. For example:

- **Memory and learning**—Memorize favorite poems or songs, learn to identify birds, or memorize new dance steps.
- **Music**—Learn to play a musical instrument.
- **Concentration**—Play computer games, chess, or bridge.
- **Planning**—Design your own website, plan a garden, or organize a fundraiser for a charity.
- **Language**—Join a book-discussion group, do crossword puzzles or word games, learn a new language.
- **Spatial relationships**—Learn to draw, take a pottery class, learn wood carving, or play board games.
- **Reaction speed and manual dexterity**—Play ping-pong, tennis, or assemble jigsaw puzzles.

Painting mental pictures can help make your memory more reliable. A small study published in June 2004 in *Psychology and Aging* found that visualizing an important health task—testing blood sugar—made older adults 50% more likely to do it the next day than those who used other memory techniques, such as verbally repeating the task in advance. Previous research has shown that the same visualization strategy also can help with everyday activities. So if there's a task you have trouble remembering, try taking a few minutes the night before to form a detailed mental movie of when, where, and how you'll get it done. (Consumer Reports Health—'"Brain workouts boost mental prowess"— closeup—"Alzheimer's: New Developments, New Hope"—Did You Know? "Visualization aids memory." *Consumer Reports*, 48, October 2004.)

For most seniors, cognitive changes are slowly progressive, the result of many factors, and not rapidly reversible. Studies suggest that daily physical and mental exercising improves mental abilities. Americans should avoid exposure to excess free radicals, which are known to increase risk of strokes, heart disease, and cancer. Lifestyle measures include consuming at least five servings of fruits and vegetables a day to decrease free radical formation in the body.

What is cognition? As defined in *Stedman's Medical Dictionary*, 27th edition, cognition includes the mental activities associated with thinking, learning, and memory. These processes should occur in the mind without conscious effort. Unfortunately, elevated blood pressure, head trauma, inadequate nutrient intake, polypharmacy, and environmental toxins can alter cognitive function in seniors.

Wearing a plain house dress and a big apron, her pockets stuffed with plastic checkers ... head down, eyes blank ... she shuffled aimlessly around the activity room. When asked to read a page from a book, the 70-year-old woman read aloud, clear as a bell. Dr. Cameron Camp, who heads the Myers Research Institute in Beachwood, Ohio, sees miracles like this day after day with Alzheimer's patients. While research typically focuses on preventing

Alzheimer's or delaying its progress in the early stages, some medical specialists and long-term care professionals are investigating activities that will help patients in the later stages.

Dr. Camp began his research 10 years ago when he observed the activities developed for young children by the educator Maria Montessori, whose method is followed today in Montessori schools around the world. Camp adapted these kinds of exercises for older people with dementia, tailoring them to the individual's background and interests. People with Alzheimer's "live in the moment, and our job is to give them as many good moments as we can," Camp says. After Alzheimer's patients were given the large-print books, many could read aloud and discuss the books. (Google: Montessori work helps elderly with dementia: Acar-Dreyer. For nine simple habits you can adopt that may delay dementia, see the September-October 2005 issue of *AARP Magazine*.)

- "Lost & Found—Promising Therapy for Alzheimer's Draws Out the Person Inside the Patient" by Barbara Basler, *AARP Bulletin,* 10, 11, 17, September 2005.
- "What You Need To Know Now," by Dr. Isadore Rosenfeld, *Parade,* 6, January 15, 2006.
- "Seniors Who Exercise Have Lower Risk for Alzheimer's" *The Oregonian,* C10, January 18, 2006.

Midway through a conversation, you lose track of the point you were trying to make. You pick up the phone at work, but can't recall the person you were going to dial. You can never seem to remember where you parked your car. You chalk up these events to senior moments, but deep down, you wonder if you're on your way to developing Alzheimer's disease.

CHAPTER 14

SUMMARY

Although you can't reverse the aging process, you can adopt strategies now that can help you prevent, or at least delay, Alzheimer's. Many of these brain-healthy habits are the same ones that help fend off other diseases, including cancer, diabetes, and cardiovascular disease.

Below are twelve strategies to help prevent Alzheimer's.

1. "Anything you can do to reduce your risk for atherosclerosis, diabetes, and stroke will also help you reduce your risk for dementia," says Todd E. Feinberg, MD, chief of the Yarmon Neurobehavior and Alzheimer's Disease Center at Beth Israel Medical Center in New York City and co-author of *What To Do When The Doctor Says It's Early-Stage Alzheimer's.*

2. Get in touch with your inner athlete. Physical activity is as good for your brain as it is for your body. "Exercise is probably the single most important thing you can do to keep your brain healthy over time," says Daniel G.

Amen, M.D., author of *Making a Good Brain Great.* Exercise improves the heart's ability to pump blood to the brain and increases oxygen and glucose delivery. Walking 20 to 30 minutes every day is one way to stay fit. Dr. Amen's favorite exercise is table tennis.

3. Eat smart. Good nutrition keeps arteries clean and maintains blood flow to the brain.

4. Taste the rainbow. Fruits high in antioxidants include blueberries, cherries, plums, and strawberries. Good veggie choices include broccoli, kale, red peppers, and spinach.

5. Eat more fish. Salmon, mackerel, tuna, and halibut are rich in omega-3 fatty acids, which have anti-inflammatory effects that may keep AD at bay. According to howtolivepast100.com, eating fish twice a week can slow the rate of cognitive decline by 13%.

6. Limit fats and cholesterol. Too much saturated fats and cholesterol clogs the arteries, including those that lead to the brain, which raises the risk of AD.

7. Go nuts. Nuts are a good source of antioxidants. They contain fat, but it's monounsaturated, the good kind.

8. A 2005 study published in the *British Medical Journal* found that people who are overweight have an increased risk of developing dementia.

9. Challenge your brain every day. Reading, visiting museums, writing a journal, and even playing board games are good ways to keep your brain active.

10. Keep your friends close. Staying involved with friends and family can stimulate your brain.

11. Ginkgo biloba and huperzine A aren't the only substances that are intriguing Alzheimer's researchers. Curcumin, a plant substance in curry, has been found to block the formation of amyloid plaque in mice.

12. Stop brain drain. Stop smoking cigarettes. Don't watch

too much television; it doesn't challenge the brain. Reduce your stress. Reduce head trauma.

("The Healthy Mind," by Winnie Yu, *Woman's Day*, 70, 73, 74, April 18, 2006)

FACTS IN BRIEF

Dr. Andrew Dillin, while he was a biologist at California's Salk Institute for Biological Studies, and researchers from neighboring Scripps Research Institute found a way of "scrubbing" the buildup of toxic (amyloid that destroys the brain. They're on the road to a new drug. "Alzheimer's Researchers Detect Molecular Cleanup Crews" by Lauran Neergaard, The Associated Press, *The Oregonian*, August, 11, 2006, A7)

Dr. Dillin is also the Howard Hughes Medical Institute (Ashburn, VA) Medical Investigator and the Thomas and Stacey Siebel Distinguished Chair in Stem Cell Research at the Department of Molecular and Cell Biology at Cal-Berkeley.

Spinal fluid assessment—Scientists are hopeful a protein pattern is an early sign of the disease. Researchers at New York's Weill Cornell Medical College discovered a pattern of 23 proteins floating in spinal fluid that, in very preliminary testing, seems to identify Alzheimer's not perfectly, but fairly accurately. ("Alzheimer's Study Finds Possible Test" by Lauran Neergaard, The Associated Press, *The Oregonian*, December 12, 2006)

In a double-blind study involving 174 subjects with mild to moderate Alzheimer's, supplementation with omega-3 fatty acids was found to significantly reduce the decline in cognitive function in those subjects with very mild AD. After 4- to 6-month studies, the authors noted: "These results suggest that patients with very mild AD may benefit from daily supplementation of omega-3 fatty acids." ("Omega 3s and Alzheimer's Disease" *Vitamin Retailer*, December 2006)

Mary Blake Carver, 55, is among the growing ranks of people in the early stages of AD, when short-term memory is patchy, organizational skills fail, attention wanders, and initiative comes and goes. But there is still a window of opportunity—maybe one year, maybe five—to reason, communicate, and go about her life with a bit of help from those around her. New York, Chicago and San Anselmo, California, have started groups where the patients lead the discussions and plan the activities. ("Early Stage Alzheimer's Patients Start to Speak Out" by Jane Gross, *New York Times News Service, The Oregonian,* April, 1, 2007, A7)

Symptoms: Symptoms may be misleading. Many drugs prescribed for the elderly can cause confusion and memory loss. Some symptoms are depression, agitation, withdrawal, insomnia, irritability, memory loss, personality change, and senility. There are two types of dementia. Primary comes on gradually, without apparent causes. Secondary comes on suddenly from brain injury, operation, drugs, or a diabetic coma and is usually reversible. Alzheimer's is primary dementia, which shows up in the brain as tangled clumps of nerve fibers and patches of disintegrated nerves in the brain.

Causes: The cause of Alzheimer's could be a genetic abnormality. When people with Down syndrome live to their 30s or 40s, some develop Alzheimer's disease. Allergies could play a role because of poor nutrition and improper digestion. Allergies cause swelling in the brain and can cause bizarre behavior. The brain is sensitive to toxins in the bloodstream that are created from auto-intoxication and constipation. Heavy metals accumulate when minerals are lacking in the body. Minerals help prevent heavy metals from accumulating. Free radicals are seen as one cause of Alzheimer's. Free radicals destroy cells, like acid burning a hole in a cell wall. When stomach acid is lacking and is neutral, it will not break down food, and malnutrition develops. It also causes toxins to accumulate and damage cells.

Nutritional therapy: Most tap water contains aluminum and other heavy metals because of acid rain in our soil that leaks into the water. Purified water is essential to prevent accumulation of toxins. Distilled water works like a magnet, leaching out toxins. Proper digestion is necessary. A change of diet is needed, with wholesome foods that contain vitamins, minerals, and enzymes. Dead food does not contain live enzymes and nutrients are destroyed. Cooking brown rice, millet, and buckwheat in a thermos will assure the B-complex vitamins remain. Salads, sprouts, and lightly steamed vegetables help. Fresh fruit and vegetable juices will provide nutrients that are easily digested and assimilated. Useful herbs include: burdock, butcher's broom, capsicum, echinacea, garlic, ginger, ginseng, ginkgo, gotu kola, He-Shou-Wu, kelp, lobelia, passionflower, pau d'arco, psyllium, and suma.

Herbal formulas: There are numerous herbal formulas that cleanse the blood, circulatory system, colon, and digestive system. Others help improve energy and stamina, bolster the immune system, brain, and nervous system, and assist with urinary health.

Vitamins, minerals, and supplements: Vitamins A, C with bioflavonoids, and E are antioxidants that can prevent free radical damage. Vitamin E helps in brain damage. B-complex vitamins are seen lacking in people with Alzheimer's. Minerals prevent toxic metals from accumulating. Selenium and zinc are essential. Iron is needed for pure blood. All minerals are necessary for a healthy body. Blue-green algae is rich in vitamins, minerals, and amino acids. CoQ10 and germanium provide oxygen to the brain. Lecithin helps clean plaque and nourish the brain. Flaxseed oil and salmon oil lower cholesterol and prevent blood clotting. ("Alzheimer's Disease" *The Encyclopedia of Natural Remedies,* by Louise Tenney, MH, pp 259-260, Woodland Publishing Inc., 1995)

Stress: Dr. Hans Selye of Montreal (1907–1982) was a Hungarian-Canadian endocrinologist who is considered the father of the stress field. He was the world's most famous authority on stress. Mental strain (exhaustion and fear) on our body will cause it to use minerals and vitamins in excess of its normal needs. The first problem to show up is arthritis. Supplements, especially the B and C vitamins, are suggested.

During a stressful event, the body releases adrenaline from the adrenal glands, the heart rate accelerates, and breathing and blood pressure increase. Then the adrenal glands release cortisol, and the body returns to normal. In people with chronic stress, too much cortisol can be released, damaging brain cells. This can affect memory. (M. Albert, PhD, professor of neurology at Johns Hopkins, co-director of Johns Hopkins Alzheimer's Disease Center)

Herbs: Ginkgo biloba extracts are the best-selling herbal medicine in Europe. This herb's restorative effects center on the brain, specifically in memory, as well as preventing strokes, acting as an antioxidant, and treating hearing disorders. Ginkgo is known in scientific circles as a nootropic, a substance that activates the intellect. (*Psychopharmacology Bulletin; Free Radical Biology and Medicine; Biochemical Pharmacology; Biochemical and Biophysical Research Communications; Journal of Pharmacy and Pharmacology; Brain Research*)

Ginkgo clinical tests at six medical centers were conducted with 309 patients having mild dementia: 120 mg of ginkgo each day revealed moderate improvement on cognitive tests. The effects were roughly comparable to those achieved with tacrine, a drug approved in 1993 as a treatment for AD. Tacrine cost four times as much as ginkgo and was far more toxic. In clinical studies, 25% of all tacrine users developed potentially dangerous liver abnormalities. (November 3, 1997, *Newsweek*) Tacrine was discontinued in the United States in 2013 as a result of safety concerns.

Passionflower can ease anxiety without severe side effects. It has been used as an anxiety-easer and sedative for centuries by native people in North, Central, and South America. The compounds in the plant, known as flavonoids and alkaloids, regulate the neurotransmitters in the nervous system that reduce anxiety. Another flavonoid called chrysin calms the central nervous system and lowers blood pressure. Clinical studies compared passionflower to oxazepam in a group suffering from general anxiety disorder. The group taking passionflower did not have the severely impaired job performance of those taking oxazepam. (Akhondzadeh S et al. Passionflower in the treatment of generalized anxiety: a pilot double-blind randomized controlled trial with oxazepam. *Journal of Clinical Pharmacy and Therapeutics* 2001 Oct; 26(5)363-7)

One last exercise to implement: A Test: Google the SAGE Alzheimer's Memory Test (Self-Administered Geocognitive Examination).

UCLA also has a memory quiz: Dementia warning signs.

PHOTOS – ARDITH

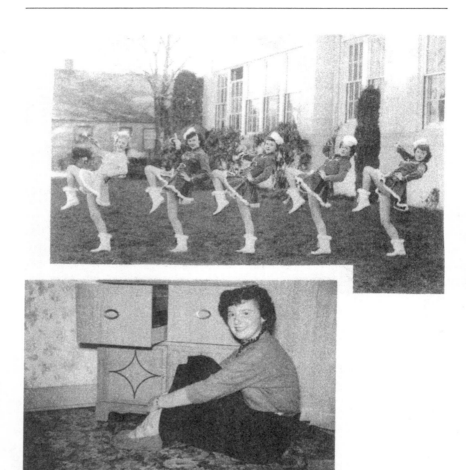

Majorette in high school – 2nd from rt.

Phonograph gift – 1951

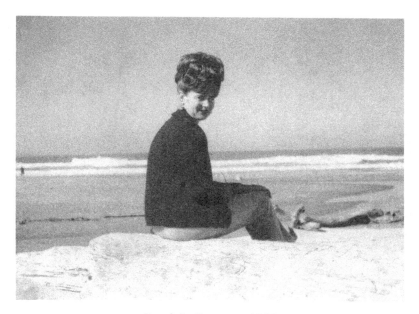

Beach in Oregon – 1966

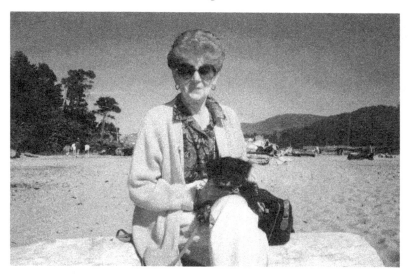

Beach in Oregon with Niko – 2004

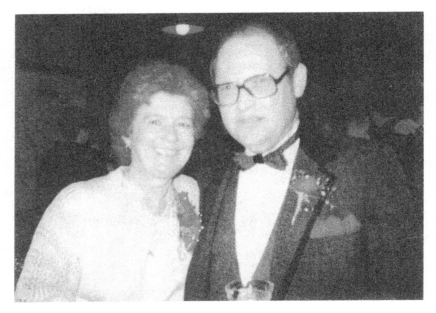

At our daughter Debbie's wedding – 1983

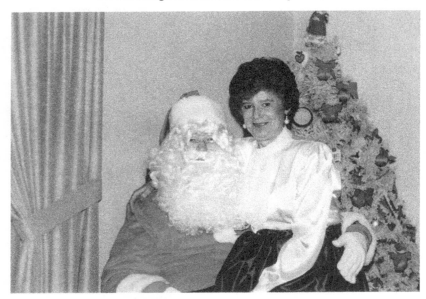

On Santa's (Matt's) lap @ Christmas

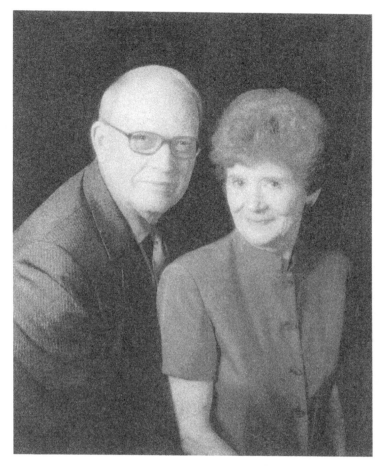

50th wedding anniversary – 2002

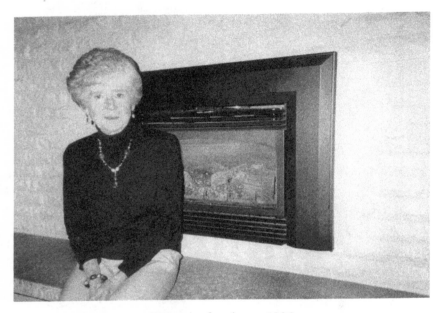

Sitting by fireplace – 1986

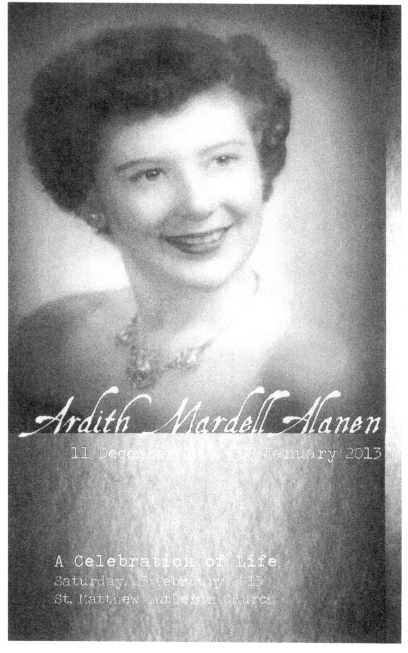

High school graduation – 1951

PHOTOS - FRED

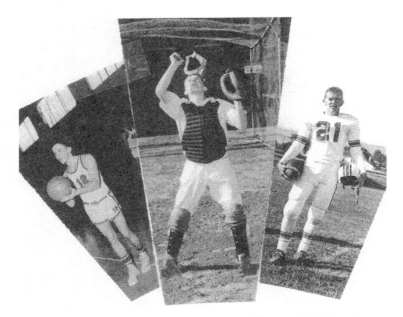

Three sport letterman in Oroville, California High School

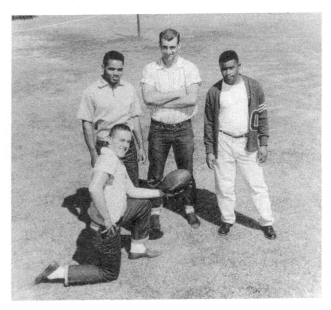

Fred with football and his backfield at Oroville Hi – State Champs

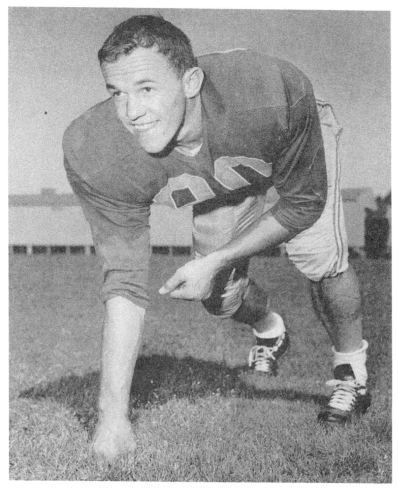

Photo shot – Yogi training as an Oregon Duck

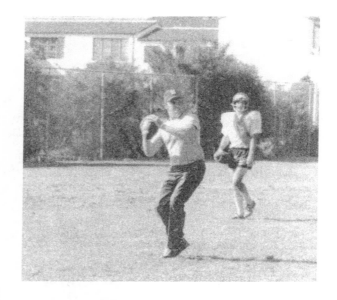

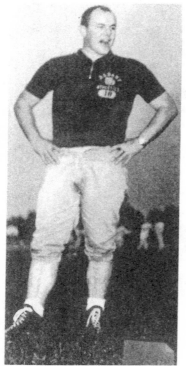

Coach Siler @ Albany High School

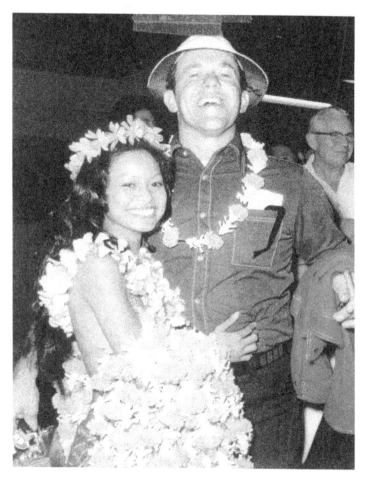

Yogi in Hawaii after a Duck football game

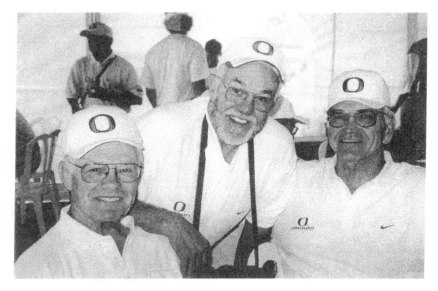

Yogi and his Oregon Ducks

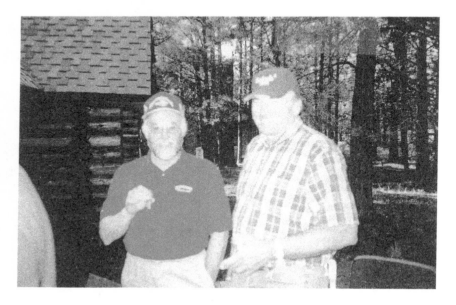

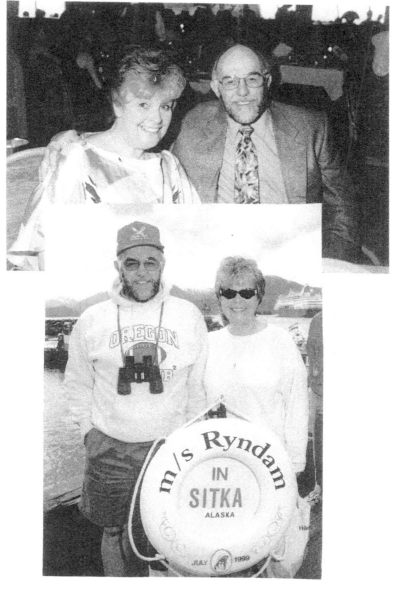

Fred and Sally

CPSIA information can be obtained
at www.ICGtesting.com
Printed in the USA
BVHW072015310120
570936BV00003B/9